Understanding the
HORSE'S
FEET

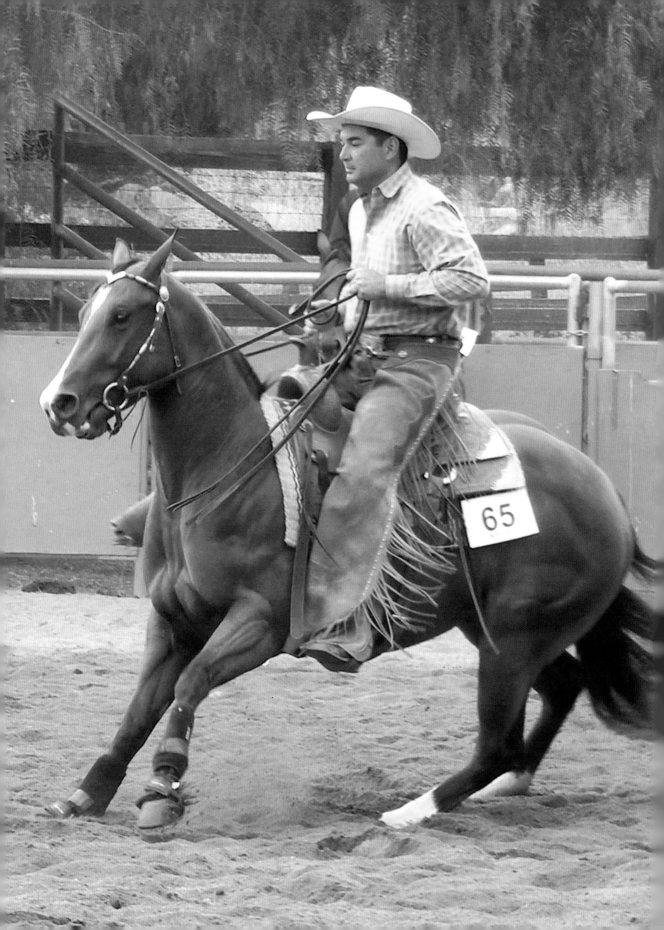

Understanding the
HORSE'S FEET

John Stewart
MA Vet, MB, MRCVS

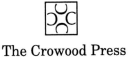

The Crowood Press

First published in 2013 by
The Crowood Press Ltd
Ramsbury, Marlborough
Wiltshire SN8 2HR

www.crowood.com

British Library Cataloguing-in-Publication Data
A catalogue record for this book is available from the British Library.

ISBN 978 1 84797 476 1

Diagrams by Charlotte Kelly

Dedication
Dedicated to Caillou, and to all the horses, ponies and donkeys that have not survived laminitis

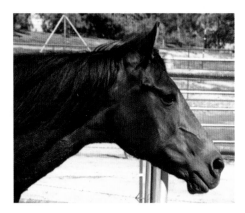

Typeset by Jean Cussons Typesetting, Diss, Norfolk

Printed and bound in India by Replika Press Pvt. Ltd.

Contents

Introduction

After I had agreed to write this book, it did not take me long to realize the enormity of the task I had set myself. I thought about the thousands of articles and hundreds of books already written about horses' feet and wondered what I could possibly contribute to the topic. I had read enough of these papers and spoken to sufficient vets, farriers and trimmers to know that there was, and still is, significant disagreement on many aspects of the horse's foot and its function – so not only was I to write on a subject where there are so many different opinions, I also had to do it in a way that would be understandable to horse owners. Yes, I panicked.

In the past, the majority of owners relied on their farrier or vet to advise them on hoof care, but nowadays, particularly with the advent of the internet, owners are doing their own research and many are becoming more proactive in the foot care of their horses. The problem for an owner is to know how much of the information available is fact, or how much might be just conjecture, and this probably applies as much to what is found in 'traditional' text books as the more speculative suggestions that circulate on some websites and internet forums. It does seem that some things have been repeated so often that they have been accepted as fact, and I find I am not the only person to question the veracity of some of these 'facts'.

Part of the fascination about horses' feet, and the problems they develop, is that there is very little that can be considered 'black' or 'white',

and there are endless shades of grey, depending on the horse, its environment, its diet or its type of work – however, this is a great part of the frustration, too. This is because something that is right for one horse might be unsuitable or impractical for another, and something that is suitable for a horse at one time may then become the wrong thing to do for it in different circumstances. Nowhere does this become more pertinent than when dealing with laminitis (*see* Chapter 7), but it applies to other situations and conditions too. Although my aim has been to provide sufficient information about the grey areas for an owner to be able, with the assistance of their hoof-care professional, to make the right decision at the right time, the book's content has been influenced by the fact that many farriers and trimmers (and vets, too) are set in their ways and tend not to be open-minded to new or different ideas. Too often I have been made aware of an owner's concerns being brushed aside, so I have felt it necessary to go into greater depth than many other 'books for owners' in the hope that a greater understanding of problems will carry more weight with these 'professionals'. I know that for many readers, parts of the book (Chapter 2, in particular) will be a challenge because they will encounter a vocabulary that is unfamiliar to them, but I believe some knowledge of the anatomy and function of the structures of the foot will help them understand the chapters that follow. If the reader is stimulated to find out more about the horse's foot, which is what I hope to achieve, understanding these terms will also help – and may even be necessary – when reading other books and articles. The areas where there is in-depth information generally cover problems or situations that an owner is more likely to be confronted with, but also topics where I have introduced some novel concepts that need an explanation. Other areas where I have provided less information may be equally important, but I have felt they were either rare conditions or ones that would necessitate direct veterinary involvement.

I may well receive criticism from some people for including some of my own theories which are the results of my research but have not been 'verified'. In the final chapter I describe the routes that my studies have taken, and the reasons for the conclusions I have come to, but because a large part of these investigations have been carried out without any fancy equipment and have mostly been from close examination of the horse's foot, I am confident that other people will find the same things, if they look.

For brevity's sake I have often used 'horse' to refer to 'horse, pony and donkey', and 'man' to include men and women. However, when it comes to foot care, my use of 'farrier' to include 'farrier, horse-shoer and foot trimmer' is perhaps more controversial. It applies to when foot balance and trimming is being discussed, since this applies to all three – though when I talk about having shoes on the feet it obviously no longer includes the barefoot trimmer. Although this book is about feet, it is vitally important not to consider them in isolation because the feet affect the rest of the horse, and the rest of the horse affects what happens to the feet. I have to confess that, whether it is a live horse, or a sculpture or a picture of one, the first things I look at are its feet; however, I do then always look at the 'whole picture' – at the beauty and the athleticism of this wonderful creature.

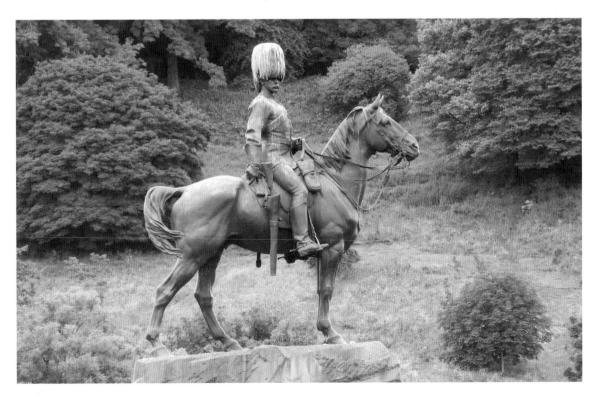

Fig. 1   Memorial to the Royal Scots Greys (1906), Princes Street, Edinburgh.

1 Evolution

If you place your hand on a table and, while leaving the finger tips in contact, raise it up until it is vertical, you will be left with just one fingernail touching the table. This illustrates the adaptive process in the horse's foot which has taken place over millions of years, starting with the horse's ancestors, Eohippus, up to the horses and ponies known collectively as Equus, which are around today.

Ancestors of the horse existed fifty million years ago, but were very different to the creature that we recognize now. Eohippus was a small hare-like animal, living and running around in swampy undergrowth on feet with four long splayed toes. As the climate changed and became drier, the swamps and forests gradually disappeared and were replaced by open plains, and Eohippus had to adapt to take advantage of this new environment in order to survive. Modifications in its tooth structure enabled it to cope with grazing pasture rather than browsing bushes, and by changing its limb structure it was better able to survive in the open ground.

The limb changes included increasing the length of the legs, which allowed these prehistoric horses to take longer strides and so enabled them to run faster to escape from predators. Part of this leg-lengthening process was achieved by raising the digits to a more upright position. In the exercise described in the first paragraph, when you raised your hand from the table, the first finger to lose contact was your thumb; this digit was in fact already absent in the Eohippus, which had only four toes – but when you raised the hand further, the little finger lost contact, and this demonstrates the adaption that occurred over twenty million years, and can be seen in the Mesohippus, which had only three toes.

In the next twenty million years the digits became even more upright, with the inside and outside toes reducing in size so that they probably only made contact in wetter ground: the horse that characterized this evolutionary stage was called the Merychippus. The Pliohippus, which lived between ten and one million years ago, had one long toe, and Equus, the modern horse, adapted further to end up moving around on its middle finger nail, the hoof. The remnants of the other two digits were retained as the splint bones, lying just to the

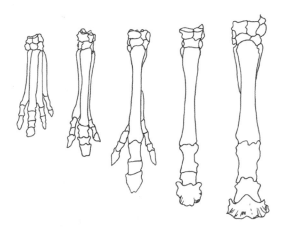

Fig. 2   The bones of the digits of 1. Eohippus, 2. Mesohippus, 3. Merychippus, 4. Pliohippus, 5. Equus.

back of the cannon bone (the third metacarpus) and acting as support to the horse's knee (the equivalent of our wrist).

The anatomy of the equine digit is somewhat different from our equivalent finger, although the basic form is similar. If, with a straight arm, you press down on your middle finger till your finger is bent back by about forty-five degrees to the perpendicular, this is the equivalent position of the horse's lower limb.

(as explained above). As the lower bones of the legs became longer, the upper bones of the limb remained short, and the heavy muscles that attach the trunk to these bones became more powerful. Reciprocal pulley systems evolved, with the arrangement of the tendons allowing the limb joints to bend or straighten together – wind resistance is reduced by the horse being able to fold the legs up under the body when he is moving at speed.

ADAPTATIONS NECESSARY FOR EOHIPPUS' SURVIVAL

So what were the adaptations required in Eohippus in order for him and his descendants to survive the change from forest to prairie? Already mentioned is the reduction in the number of digits, with more toes being of benefit in marshy ground, but a single one being better for firmer ground. However, in order to survive, these prehistoric horses also needed stamina to endure the long migrations required to find food and water, and the ability to remain standing a lot of the time in an energy-efficient way.

The Requirement for Speed

The speed of movement of an animal depends on the length and frequency of its stride: the longer and quicker the stride, the faster the animal will go. As well as lengthening the lower bones of the limbs and adopting a more upright posture, an increase in stride length in the horse was achieved by an evolutionary change which resulted in the loss of the clavicle (collar bone), thereby allowing a greater range of movement of the shoulder.

An increase in stride frequency was achieved as a result of a number of evolutionary changes, which included the reduction in weight of the lower limb by reducing the number of digits

The Requirement for Stamina

The stamina required for long migrations was improved by evolving with 'energy-efficient motion'. The tendons and ligament that support the fetlock joint – the 'suspensory apparatus' – evolved to be better able to store energy, to act like a spring, and as the leg bones became longer, so too did the tendons, to produce larger 'springs'. This reduces the energy required by the muscles when the horse moves, allowing it to travel further with less effort.

The Requirement to Save Energy while Standing

As the horse evolved to be a plains-living animal, it increasingly relied on flight to escape from predators, and it was therefore important that it stayed on its feet to enable a quick getaway. It developed mechanisms to enable it to rest whilst standing: these are referred to as its 'stay apparatus'. This describes the system of ligaments in the horse's legs, which help to support it when it is standing, so that it can maintain the limb joints extended with minimal energy use. It can also 'lock' the patella (the knee-cap) in the hind legs, and has supporting ligaments to the superficial and deep digital flexor tendons – the superior and inferior 'check' ligaments – which allow the muscles to relax while tension is maintained in the tendons, thus conserving energy.

EQUUS

Along with our domesticated horses, ponies and donkeys, the species Equus includes the zebra, wild asses, and the only species of wild horse surviving, the Mongolian wild horse, or Przewalski's horse, named after the Russian explorer who discovered it. These horses would be extinct in the wild were it not for breeding programmes in zoos which have allowed their reintroduction to Central Asia, and the re-establishment of a viable population.

Man has only been involved in the selective breeding of horses within the past three and a half thousand years, since they were first domesticated, thereby producing the diverse range of breeds that we see today. Initially, domesticated horses were used for work and war, but whereas the donkey is still used in many countries as a 'beast of burden', the role of the horse has changed, and in most countries it is now mainly used for pleasure, and often in the pursuit of sports.

Selective breeding has produced stronger animals to cope with the 'unnatural' situation of carrying a rider, but by breeding for certain sporting requirements, some other, more detrimental, characteristics have been perpetuated. At the individual level,

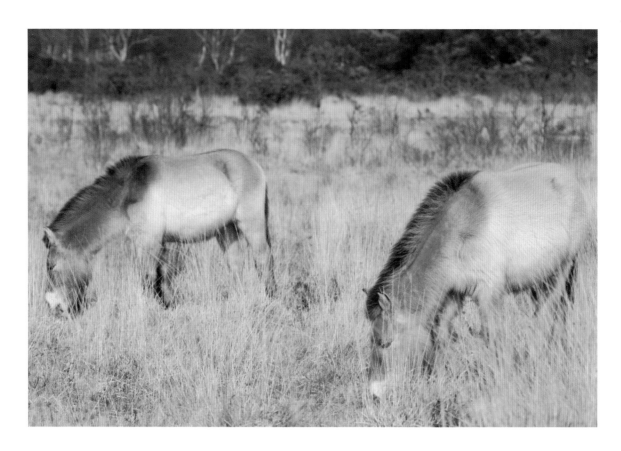

Fig. 3   Two young Przewalski stallions – part of the conservation programme at Marwell Wildlife, Hampshire, UK (Photo courtesy of Martin Wilkie).

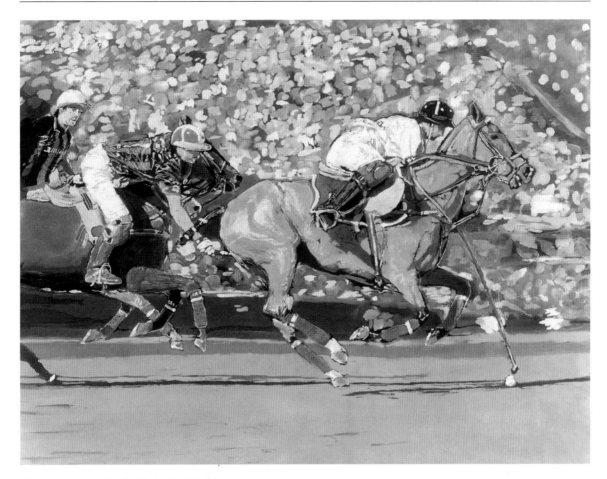

Fig. 4   The Finals – batik by Rosi Robinson.

many are bred for sentimental reasons or financial gain, rather than concentrating on producing offspring of better structural quality. Unfortunately, man has also significantly altered the lifestyle for these domesticated horses, away from the environment in which they evolved to survive. Providing a diet that is often far removed from the foodstuffs and forage that would be available in the wild, and limiting the horse's opportunity to satisfy its innate requirement for movement, has resulted in changed metabolic processes in its body, and in particular in its feet – which is the aspect of greater interest to us.

2 The Structure and Anatomy of the Foot

Although this book is about the horse's feet, it is vitally important not to consider them in isolation because the feet affect the rest of the horse, and the rest of the horse affects what happens to the feet. Because a horse's weight is distributed between its four limbs, and it is the four feet that have to carry it all, the greatest challenge to the foot is how to deal with the forces of impact and weight-bearing. The foot is generally able to withstand these forces because all the structures in it play their part in absorbing or spreading these forces – these include:

- Laminae (stretch)
- Hoof capsule (change of shape)
- Sole (stretching and flattening)
- Circulation (hydraulic response)
- Bone (minimal)
- Articular cartilage (compression)

- Ligaments (stretch)
- Tendons (stretch)
- Frog (compression)
- Digital cushion (compression)
- Collateral cartilages (load redistribution)

Although this chapter may appear challenging for readers as they are introduced to an unfamiliar vocabulary, some knowledge of the anatomy of the different structures in the horse's foot will give an insight into how the foot copes with these forces, and I hope will help the reader better understand the chapters that follow.

THE PROPERTIES OF BONE

Bones must be strong enough to support the weight of the body; they must be big enough – have a large enough surface area – to

---

STRUCTURAL PROTEINS IN THE BODY

Collagen is a protein made up of chains of amino acids that bind together to form strong, inelastic fibres. Collagen forms a structural matrix that gives tissues their shape and provides them with strength. Over a quarter of the total body protein is collagen.

Elastin is similar to collagen but gets elastic properties from the way the units bind together to produce branching fibres.

Fibroblasts are the cells that produce these fibrous proteins as well as the other constituents (glycoproteins) that make up the tissues that surround them (the extracellular matrix).

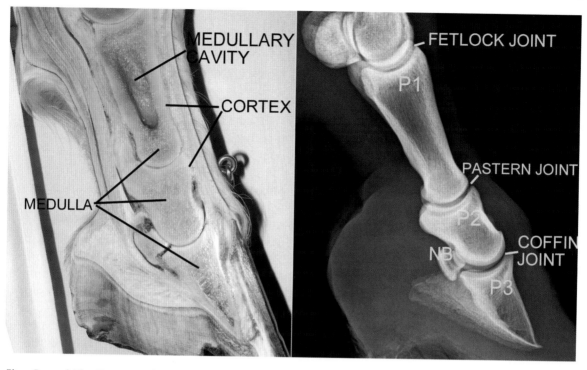

Figs. 5a and 5b   Denser and thicker bone shows up as the brighter white areas on the radiograph. The outer part of the bone is made up of dense cortex and inside this is the network of trabeculae that makes up the 'spongy' bone of the medulla. The bone ends are kept apart in the joints by articular cartilage, which does not show up on radiographs.

support soft tissue attachments; and they must be light enough in weight to reduce inertia – to minimize the effort required for rapid movement of the legs.

Bones are rigid structures with minerals laid down on a collagen matrix. Without the collagen framework, bones would be extremely brittle and very liable to break, and without the mineral deposits they would bend and be unable to support weight.

Bone status varies during the life of the horse, with less density both early and later in life. The developing bones of foals are more pliable because they contain less mineral (mineral to matrix 35 per cent: 65 per cent) than is present in adult bone (65 per cent: 35 per cent); in the old horse, the mineral content of bone tends to decrease, resulting in some reduction in bone density.

Completely solid bones would be stronger, but the greater weight would make it far more difficult for the muscles to move the limbs, so there has to be some compromise between strength and weight of bone. Bones have an outer layer of dense compact bone (cortex) and a core made up of a honeycomb-like network of bone (trabeculae), sometimes referred to as 'spongy' bone. The compact bone over the joint surface is thin, but particularly dense and smooth. Spongy bone completely fills the core of shorter bones, but in longer bones is limited to each end, and the space in the middle (the medullary cavity) contains blood-producing cells, known as bone marrow.

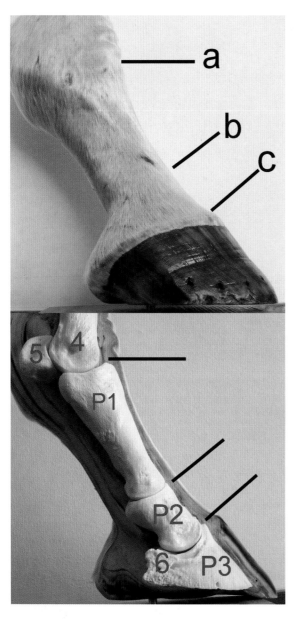

Figs. 6 and 6b   P1, P2 and P3 = the three phalangeal bones of the digit; 4 = cannon bone; 5 = proximal sesamoid bone; 6 = navicular bone (not visible – hidden behind palmar process of P3). Black lines to a) fetlock; b) pastern; c) coffin joints.

of the horse as well as the tension from the attached ligaments and tendons. Bones are able to withstand the very large compressive forces that are applied along their length, but are less able to cope with forces in other directions, which make them liable to fracture.

Rather than the inert object we see in a dried skeleton, bone is a living tissue that has bone formation and remodelling going on all the time. Bones are covered by periosteum, a fibrous sheet of collagen that has small blood vessels and nerve endings and a population of cells involved in the production of bone (osteoblasts) and in its breakdown (osteoclasts). The balance of activity of these two types of cell can be seen in physiological processes (normal functioning of bone) as well as pathological ones (arising from disease). The response of bone when subjected to the increased forces from exercise is to increase osteoblast activity, which thickens cortical bone and remodels the trabeculae in spongy bone, to change alignment and strengthen the bone along the lines of stress.

In some pathological processes, bone remodels in response to pressure, which is seen most commonly in the foot with the change in shape of the tip of P3 (coffin bone) in chronic laminitis.

THE ANATOMY OF THE LIMB BONES

The bones of the horse's limbs are similar to those of many other mammals, but have developed their own special features. You may find it helpful to compare their bones and joints to your own.

The Bones of the Digit

Starting from the bottom, the bones from the horse's foot to his fetlock are equivalent to those

The thickness and distribution of the two types of bone are arranged to withstand the stresses and strains that act on the individual bone – the lines of pressure from the weight

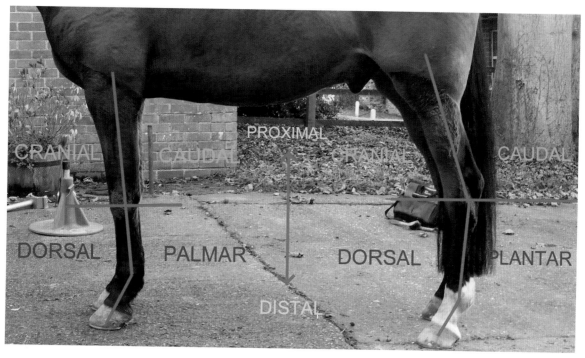

Fig. 7 *Terms used to describe the positions of structures on a horse's legs: 'palmar' is to the back of the front leg ('plantar' for the hind leg), 'proximal' is when something is higher on the leg and closer to the body.*

of our middle finger (or middle toe), and are the three bones of the digit. These bones are referred to by several names, but most simply as P3, which is enclosed inside the hoof (end of the finger, with nail), P2 (the middle bone) and P1 (the third finger bone) – *see* synopsis below. The same names are used for the bones of the digit in the hind foot.

P3 = P III = third phalanx = distal phalanx = coffin bone = pedal bone
P2 = P II = second phalanx = middle phalanx = short pastern bone
P1 = P I = first phalanx = proximal phalanx = long pastern bone

The Distal Phalanx [P3]

P3 is an irregularly shaped bone with three surfaces and three borders and enclosed entirely within the hoof capsule (*see* Fig 8).

The 'dorsal surface' of P3 is the outer surface of the bone to which the hoof is attached. The articular surface is covered by cartilage and is where P2 and the navicular bone make contact with it in the coffin joint. The 'palmar surface' is the underside of the bone and includes the smooth 'solar surface' that is covered by the sole, and a roughened posterior rim, the 'flexor surface', where the tendon of the deep flexor muscle attaches.

The central prominence on the top of the bone, on the proximal border, is the 'extensor process', where the common digital extensor tendon attaches. The 'palmar processes' are the 'wings' of P3 and extend backwards (palmarly) from the base of the bone.

The periosteum of P3 appears to be more disorganized and less distinct than that of other bones, and this is attributed to the particular stresses it is subjected to. Between the periosteum and the hoof is an even layer

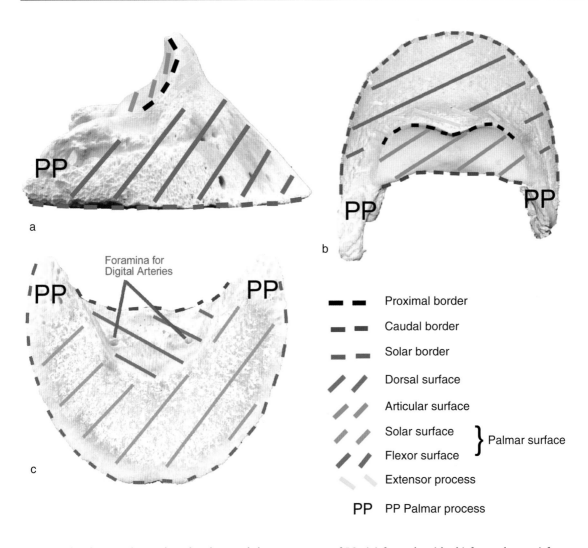

Fig. 8 *The three surfaces, three borders and three processes of P3: (a) from the side; b) from above; c) from underneath.*

of tissue (dermis), which has an intricate network of collagen fibres, blood vessels and sensory nerve endings. With its tough fibrous attachments to the hoof (laminae) and the bone (periosteum), it provides a very strong connection for the two structures. The result is that in a normal foot, the dorsal hoof wall and the dorsal surface of P3 remain parallel to each other, and the forces acting on the bone are transmitted evenly to the hoof wall and vice versa. Likewise, the sole follows the concave shape of the underside of the bone because of the even layer of tissue connecting it to the solar surface of the bone.

The Sesamoid Bones

The horse has additional bones called sesamoid bones, which reduce friction and change the

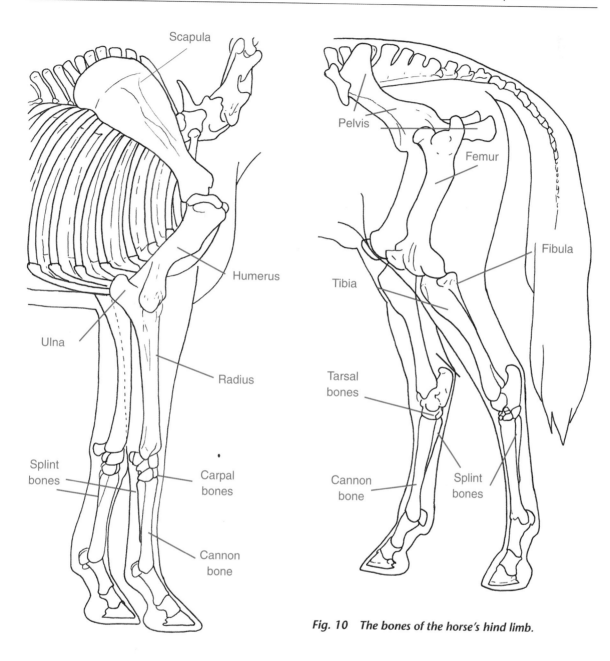

Scapula

Humerus

Ulna

Radius

Splint
bones

Carpal
bones

Cannon
bone

Fig. 9   The bones of the horse's forelimb.

Pelvis

Femur

Fibula

Tibia

Tarsal
bones

Cannon
bone

Splint
bones

Fig. 10   The bones of the horse's hind limb.

direction of pull of the flexor tendons as they pass over the back (palmar) surface of the fetlock and coffin joints. The two proximal (higher) **sesamoid bones** are often referred to simply as the sesamoid bones, whereas the distal (lower) sesamoid bone is far more commonly called the **navicular bone**. (We

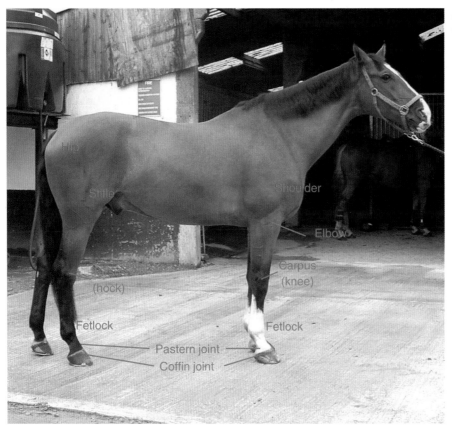

Fig. 11 The limb joints of the horse.

have the equivalent of the proximal sesamoid bones at the base of our thumb and big toe.)

The Limb Bones

In the horse, the equivalent of the five metacarpal bones of our hands, connecting our fingers to our wrist, or the metatarsal bones between our toes and ankle, have been reduced to the one long weight-bearing bone, the cannon bone, with the remnants of the second and fourth becoming the splint bones.

In the foreleg the horse's 'knee' is the carpus, the equivalent of our wrist, and is made up of a complex arrangement of two layers of small bones. In our forearm we have two bones, the radius and the ulna, that give us the ability to

turn our hand over. The weight-bearing horse's limb requires far greater stability, and although both the radius and ulna, with the lower (distal) end of the humerus, make up the horse's elbow joint (the same as ours), the ulna reaches only half way down the back of the radius, leaving only the one bone in the horse's forearm that is joined to the knee (carpus).

In the horse's hind leg, the complex joint at the proximal end (top) of the cannon bone is the tarsus, commonly referred to as the hock, and the equivalent of the ankle in our human leg. Between our ankle and knee – the hock and the stifle in the horse – the major weight-bearing bone is the tibia; the accompanying fibula has a minor role in our ankle joint, but no involvement in the horse's hock, remaining only as a very small remnant to the side of the tibia.

JOINTS

If bone were to contact bone in a joint, the structure would have very little or no concussion-absorbing properties and the ends of the bones would very rapidly be destroyed. To allow the joint to absorb concussion and to reduce friction within it, the ends of the bones are covered by cartilage, and the joint space between them is filled with fluid.

The joint capsule that surrounds a joint has two layers: a tough outer fibrous membrane and an inner synovial membrane, which produces the synovial fluid that provides shock absorption and decreases friction in the moving joint.

The Joints of the Lower Limb

The joints in the horse's lower limb – and therefore the ones most closely related to the foot – are the coffin joint, the pastern joint and the fetlock joint; they are further identified as follows:

The coffin joint: The distal interphalangeal joint (DIPJ), involving P2, P3 and the navicular bone (described in more detail below).

The pastern joint: The proximal interphalangeal joint, that involves P1 and P2.

The fetlock joint: This refers to the metacarpo-phalangeal joint in the foreleg, and the metatarso-phalangeal joint in the hind leg; it involves the cannon bone, P1 and the proximal sesamoid bones.

The shape of the fetlock, pastern and coffin joints allows significant movement in one direction, which is backwards and forwards in the sagittal plane (in the line of the body). This is very important for an animal running at speed over uneven ground, particularly for one

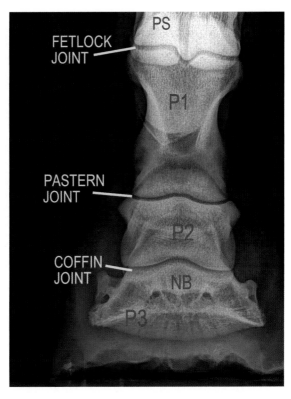

Fig. 12 Radiograph (DP view) showing the joints of the digit. The shapes of the bones help to limit the direction of movement. Articular cartilage does not show up on radiographs, so appears as dark lines between the bones. PS = proximal sesamoid, NB = navicular bone.

the size of a horse. The direction of movement is limited by matching curves and ridges on the joint surfaces of the bones, with the joints relying on ligaments and tendons to maintain them within safe working limits. The elbow, stifle, carpus and tarsus are more complex joints, but the alignment of the bones and the way they fit together also limits their movement to the sagittal plane.

A joint functions best when the load on it is spread evenly over the joint surfaces. At the gallop, when the horse tucks its legs up

DEFINITIONS RELATING TO JOINT MOVEMENT

Flexion: The bending of a joint, when the angle between the two bones is reduced.

Extension: The opposite of flexion, when the joint is straightened and there is an increase in angle between the bones.

Dorsal flexion (or overextension): When the angle between the bones diminishes again after extension of the joint moves the bones beyond a straight line; an obvious example of this is the fetlock joint in the horse's normal stance position.

Hyperflexion and hyperextension: Generally refer to when the joint is flexed or extended beyond its normal limits, resulting in damage to the joint structures.

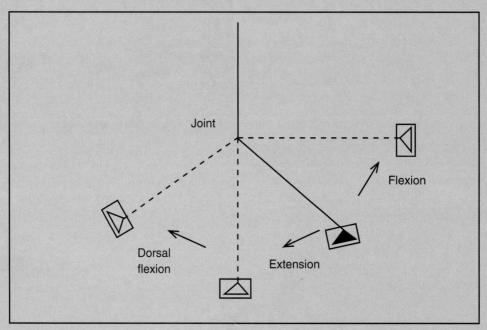

Fig. 13 Joint movement.

under its body, the uneven (asymmetrical) shape of some joints means that the opposing bones will move in a slightly different plane; however, when the horse takes weight on the bones, they all need to be aligned in order to provide maximum stability. Changes in a horse's weight-bearing position due to uneven ground, imbalance of the feet, or a change in action from lameness elsewhere, can load joints unevenly, putting increased strain on their supporting structures.

The Coffin Joint

The lowest joint of the leg is the coffin (distal

interphalangeal) joint, involving P2 and P3, with the load from P2 (the weight of the horse) being spread by the inclusion of the navicular bone in this joint.

The area of articular contact of the bones in the coffin joint is enclosed inside the hoof, but the joint capsule that surrounds it extends above the hoof wall at the front of the pastern. This is the common site for sampling joint fluid, to identify joint disease, or for giving injections into the joint. The palmar pouch, at the back of the coffin joint, is also accessible, and is the route commonly used for examining the joint by arthroscopy (*see* Fig. 15).

The front and back surfaces of the navicular bone lie within different synovial sacs. The dorsal (front) surface of the navicular bone that articulates with P2 and P3 is in the coffin joint, whereas its palmar (back) surface is in the navicular bursa. On one side, the synovial fluid helps to lubricate the articular cartilage in the joint, and on the other side helps the deep digital flexor tendon to slide over the palmar surface of the navicular bone. The complex arrangement of ligaments supporting the navicular bone will be discussed when considering navicular disease in Chapter 11.

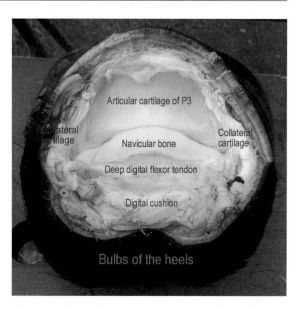

Fig. 14   The coffin joint exposed by the removal of P2 in a hoof specimen (seen from above). The articular (joint) cartilage of P3 and the navicular bone, seen as light blue areas on image, but glistening white in life.

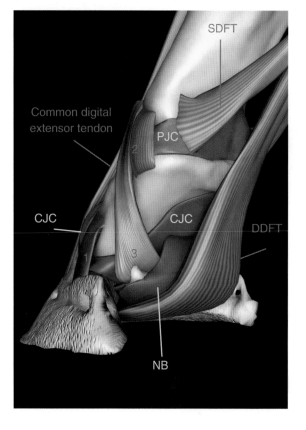

Fig. 15   The supporting structures of the pastern and coffin joints.
(PJC = pastern joint capsule, and CJC = the coffin joint capsule – in brown)
1 = collateral ligament of the coffin joint (P3 & P2)
2 = collateral ligament of pastern joint (P2 & P1)
3 = the vertical branch of the navicular suspensory ligament (navicular bone to P1)
Common digital extensor tendon inserting on the extensor process of P3.
DDFT = the deep digital flexor tendon
SDFT = the superficial digital flexor tendon
NB = navicular bursa
(Image: Science in 3D, University of Georgia Research Foundation)

LIGAMENTS

The largest ligament in the leg is the suspensory ligament, which supports the fetlock when this joint is in dorsal flexion. The suspensory ligament and the two digital flexor tendons make up the 'suspensory apparatus', and will be discussed together later.

As well as the suspensory ligament, there are two other forms of ligament that provide stability to the lower joints of the leg. There are strong fibrous bands close to the joints that attach the ends of the bones to each other, positioned in a way that limits the range of movement. These are the lateral and medial collateral ligaments of the joints, and they generally have a close association with the joint capsule. There are also three broader ligaments, known as annular ligaments, which are made up of a meshwork of fibres and are more superficial, lying just beneath the skin: they cradle the fetlock, the pastern joint and the coffin joint, supporting them and maintaining the position of the tendons as they cross them.

Although the ligaments in the foot primarily help to maintain flexion and extension of the coffin joint , they do have to allow this joint more lateral movement to compensate as a horse travels over uneven surfaces, or to cope with imbalances due to conformation. Their position and strength limit this, and their elasticity quickly returns the bones to their correct anatomical relationship when the weight is taken off the leg and in readiness for the next footfall.

TENDONS (AND MUSCLES)

Tendons are the fibrous bands that attach the ends of muscles to bones, and act as pulleys to straighten (extend) and bend (flex) joints that they cross when the muscle contracts. There are no muscles below the knee or hock in the

horse, and movement of the lower limb joints is the result of the pull on the long tendons, inserting on the phalangeal bones (P1, P2 and P3), from muscles that originate above the knee and hock.

'Origin' and 'insertion' are terms used to describe the two areas of attachment of ligaments and of muscles via their tendons. In the limb, 'origin' refers to the proximal (closer to the body) attachment of a muscle or ligament, and 'insertion' applies to its distal attachment (further from the body.)

Tendons are made up of bundles of collagen fibres that give them great tensile strength, and each complete tendon unit is covered by a tough membrane, the tendon sheath. Even though they contain little elastin, tendons do have elastic properties and are able to 'store energy' when stretched. The fibres of collagen, and the glycoproteins that make up the tendon, deform when put under tension, allowing the tendon to stretch. The energy input that causes this is released when tension is removed, as the collagen and glycoproteins return to their resting state.

Muscles contract in response to motor nerve stimuli, with active shortening of the muscle units, but there is no active process that lengthens them, and they have to rely on the contraction of muscles with an opposing action to be able to lengthen when they relax (are no longer stimulated). Joints have one or more muscles that cause them to extend, and one or more muscles that result in flexion when they contract.

The muscles involved in the flexion and the extension of the fetlock, pastern and coffin joints are identified, with the suspensory ligament, in Fig. 16. Of the four muscles, only the tendons of the common digital extensor (on the extensor process) and the deep digital flexor (on the flexor surface) insert on P3.

The deep digital flexor tendon (DDFT), as well as flexing the coffin joint, plays a significant role in stabilizing it when weight is put on the foot,

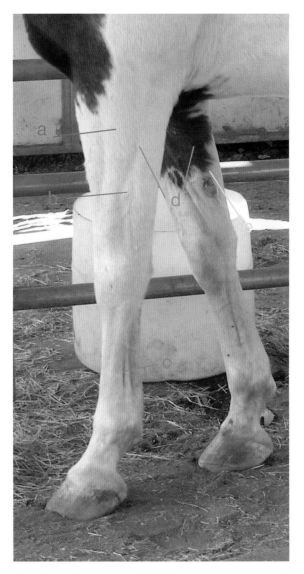

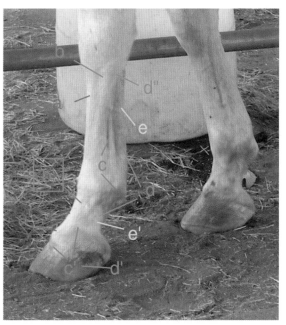

Figs. 16a and 16b   Muscles and tendons that extend and flex the digit, plus the suspensory ligament a. Common digital extensor (CDE) muscle and tendon. a'. The tendon inserts on P1, P2 and the extensor process of P3; b. Lateral digital extensor muscle and tendon. Its position is mostly deep to CDE. b'. The tendon inserts on P1; c. The suspensory ligament originates from the back of the cannon. It divides to insert on each proximal sesamoid bone. At the level of the sesamoids, c'. An extensor branch passes dorsally to join the CDE tendon, and a second branch inserts on the sesamoid bone, and then on to P1 (not shown); d. Deep digital flexor muscle and tendon. The muscle is deep to the muscles that flex the knee, with only the part of the muscle originating on the back of the elbow that can be palpated directly. d'. The tendon (DDFT) inserts on the caudal border of P3. d". is the site of the supporting ligament of the DDFT, the inferior check ligament; e. Superficial digital flexor muscle and tendon. The muscle is also deep to flexor muscles of the knee, but can be palpated to the medial side at the back of the leg. e'. The tendon (SDFT) inserts on the palmar surface of P2 and P1.

by providing support to the navicular bone that lies above (dorsal to) it in the foot. However, its supporting role is not limited to just the coffin joint: it also contributes to the stability of the entire distal limb by helping to prevent hyperextension of the fetlock and pastern joints, as well as providing support behind the knee.

The suspensory ligament divides twice at its lower (distal) end, firstly to attach to each sesamoid bone and from there to insert on P1, but also a branch passes forwards on each side of the pastern to join to the common digital extensor tendon (*see* Fig. 16). Because of the position of the DDFT, the SDFT and

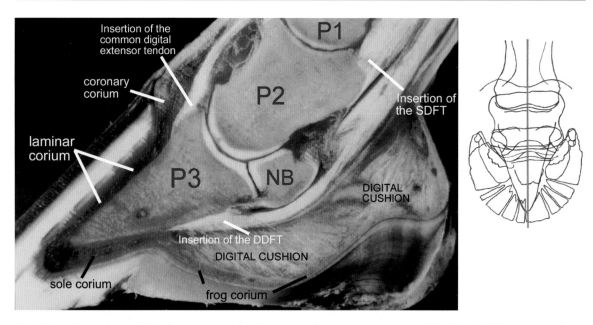

Fig. 17a *The common digital extensor tendon inserts on the extensor process of P3. The DDFT inserts on the flexor surface of P3 and the SDFT inserts on P2 and P1. The dermis of the different horn structures is often referred to as 'corium'. Blue latex has been injected into the veins of this specimen. Sagittal (midline) section of foot.* **Fig. 17b** *The position of the cut. (Image J-M. Denoix,* **The Equine Distal Limb***)*

the suspensory ligament down the back of the leg, and where they insert, dorsal flexion of the fetlock puts them under tension and causes them to stretch when weight is put on the leg.

Tendons generally become stretched when the muscle they are connected to contracts and the joint they move is under load, but this can also occur due to mechanical stretching of the muscle-tendon unit. The greatest tension occurs in a tendon when both of these forces are acting together, and this is the case for the long flexor tendons of the distal limb. When stretched, the two tendons and the suspensory ligament act like three very thick elastic bands, releasing the stored energy to help straighten the fetlock and flex the digit as weight is transferred to the opposite leg. Because of the dorsal flexion of the fetlock joint, the forces on the DDFT increase as the limb is weighted, and

with the foot on the ground, will be stretched further as the deep flexor muscle contracts in preparation for breaking-over and lifting the leg. As weight is transferred forwards to the toe, the 'recoil' from the stretched tendons helps the foot to push off from the ground prior to flexion of the leg.

Although modern running shoes may have changed the way some people run, those who run barefoot do so on the ball of the foot, making use of the stretch of the tendons to provide a more comfortable landing and to benefit from the tendon recoil as they push off.

THE COLLATERAL CARTILAGES OF THE FOOT

Also referred to as the ungular or lateral

cartilages, the collateral cartilages are a pair of rhomboid-shaped (a sloping rectangle) plates of cartilage that are attached to the palmar processes of P3, on each side of the foot. They provide a surface for the attachment of the hoof in areas where there is no bone for it to attach to. They are mostly enclosed within the hoof with their shape following the curve of the hoof wall, but the thinner proximal (top) edge can be palpated through the skin above the hoof wall. Ligaments connect the collateral cartilages to most of the other foot structures, including P3, P2, P1, the navicular bone, the DDFT and also, at their base, to the opposite cartilage.

The collateral cartilages of young horses are generally very similar in shape and structure regardless of breed, but their form is found to vary in older horses. This is due to the addition of variable amounts of fibrocartilage to their inner surface. As more fibrocartilage is laid down, it incorporates the network of veins in the area and infiltrates the structure of the digital cushion (*see* below) between the collateral cartilages. The addition of this fibrocartilage is considered to be a positive feature in a foot.

In the older horse it is common to find some degree of calcification of the collateral cartilages, referred to as 'sidebone'. Starting from the base of the collateral cartilages, bone cells (osteoblasts) infiltrate the cartilage to lay down bone, and this is seen on radiographs as extensions to the palmar processes of P3.

The role of the collateral cartilages, by connecting to all the surrounding structures, is to maintain the anatomical relationship of these structures and to spread the forces they are subjected to. The collateral cartilages are involved in the expansion of the hoof, when P2 descends into the hoof capsule forcing the cartilages out when weight is applied to the foot.

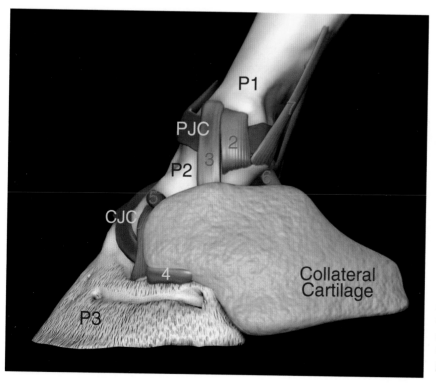

Fig. 18 A collateral cartilage is closely associated with each of the palmar processes of P3. (1) and (2) are the collateral ligaments, (3) the navicular suspensory ligament, (4), (5) and (6) are the ligaments attaching the collateral cartilage to P3 and P2. (7) is the palmar ligament between P1 and P2 (there are two pairs of palmar ligaments that help to limit over-extension of the pastern joint).

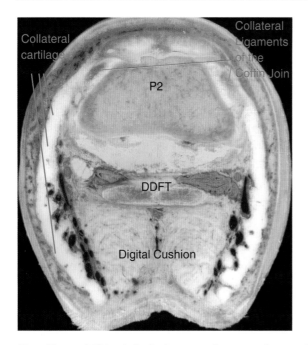
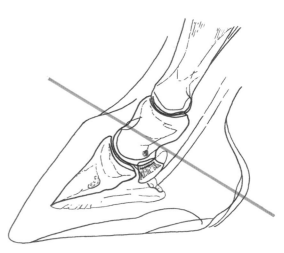

Figs. 19a and 19b   Left: Cadaver specimen cut close to the coronary band, showing the extent of the collateral cartilages. Coloured latex has been injected into veins (dark blue), arteries (red), coffin joint (yellow) and the navicular bursa (green). (Courtesy J-M. Denoix **The Equine Distal Limb***) Right: The position of the transection (cut). (Courtesy Denoix)*

The Digital Cushion

The digital cushion can be palpated as the soft structure at the back of the foot above the heels. It is made up of a network of collagen and elastin fibres surrounded by glycoproteins and some adipose tissue (fat). In some feet, fibrocartilage develops in the digital cushion, and if extensive, can provide additional support for the navicular bone. Fibrocartilage is believed to be laid down on the collateral cartilages and in the digital cushion in response to stimulation,

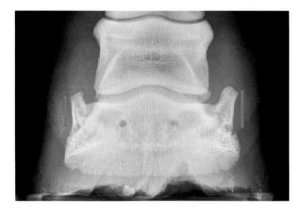

Fig. 20   Calcification of the collateral cartilages (side-bone) can be seen on radiographs, attached to the palmar processes of P3.

from ground contact of the back part of (palmar) the foot, and is absent, or limited, in feet that do not have this stimulus.

From its structure, the presumption would be that the digital cushion helps absorb the forces of concussion, but its role is less clear following the finding that there is negative pressure in it during the early/mid part of the stance phase, when the foot is beginning to take full weight. This means that compression of the frog and digital cushion can only play a part in hoof expansion late in the stance phase.

THE CIRCULATORY SYSTEM

All tissues need oxygen to survive, and they receive this, and the nutrients they require, in blood pumped out from the heart via the arterial system; waste products are returned to the heart via the venous system, with the site of transfer of nutrients and waste occurring in the capillaries.

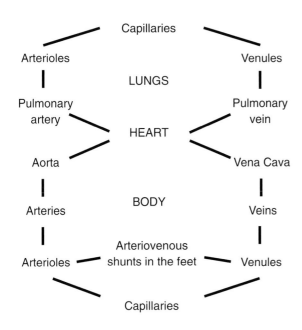

Fig. 21   The circulatory system.

When the muscles of the heart contract (systole), blood is forced through the arteries and oxygenated, nutrient-rich fluid is forced out of the capillaries into the tissues to reach the cells. Fluid returns to the bloodstream with the waste products from the chemical breakdown of the nutrients that occurred in the tissue cells. There is a relatively small negative pressure produced in the veins when the heart muscles relax (in diastole), to draw the fluid back from the tissues, and a combination of factors is required to return this into the veins and then back to the heart. Fluid returns to the capillaries by osmosis, a process whereby fluid is drawn back through a semi-permeable membrane (the capillary walls) from the surrounding tissues to equalize the concentration/dilution on the two sides. The blood cells and larger proteins are unable to pass through the capillary wall and are retained in the capillaries, and at the venous end of the capillaries, fluid is drawn back into the bloodstream to 'dilute' the concentration of these proteins.

Osmosis returns the fluid into the venous system, but the relatively small negative pressure during diastole would be insufficient to overcome the effect of gravity without further assistance. This is provided by the compression and decompression of the foot that mechanically pumps blood up the legs when the horse moves, assisted by the presence of valves in the veins which prevent back-flow.

The body also relies on a system of lymphatic vessels that it uses to remove excess interstitial fluid (fluid outside the blood vessels), at the same time passing it through lymph glands that are packed with white cells (protective cells). The thin-walled tubes of the lymphatic system are also reliant on external forces to pump the lymphatic fluid back to the heart, and they too have valves to assist this. The lymphatic system acts as a filtration system for the body.

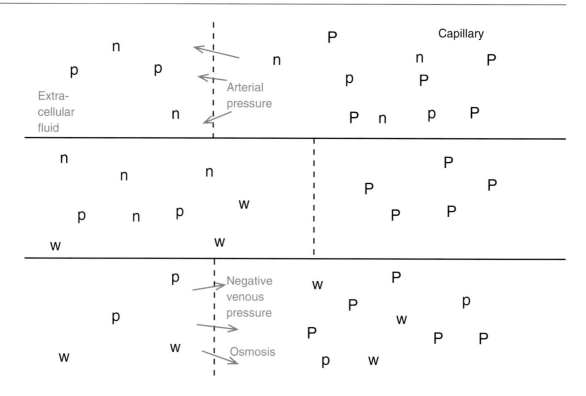

Fig. 22   Fluid is forced out of the capillary due to arterial pressure, taking with it nutrients (n) and small proteins (p). Large proteins (P) cannot pass through and are retained in the capillary. Osmosis – fluid passes through a semi-permeable membrane (capillary wall) to try to equalize concentration between the two sides. At the venous end of the capillary, fluid returns to the blood stream due to the negative pressure when the heart dilates (diastole) and from osmosis, carrying waste products (w) with it in the process.

Some people talk about the horse having 'five hearts', referring to the effect of movement on the four feet providing support for the heart, by improving blood circulation in the foot and helping pump blood and lymph back up the limbs. When any of the mechanisms for returning blood to the heart is impaired, fluid will collect in the tissues and will result in the legs becoming swollen (*see* Chapter 9).

Tissues that require more oxygen and nutrients in order to function properly have larger numbers of arteries to supply them, a greater network of capillaries to 'feed' the tissue cells, and more veins to carry away the waste products. Metabolically active tissues – for example the internal organs, the brain, muscle, and the dermis of the skin and foot – require a good blood supply, whereas tissues that rely on the physical properties of their metabolically inactive fibrous protein matrix to function – for example tendons and ligaments – have relatively few blood vessels.

The Distribution of Veins, Arteries and Nerves

There would be little to gain by providing a complete anatomical description of the

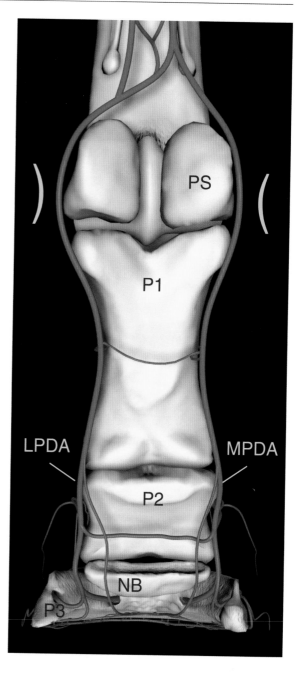

Fig. 23 *Distribution of the arterial supply to the lower leg (the veins and nerves follow a similar route). LPDA = lateral palmar digital artery, MPDA = medial palmar digital artery. Bones marked in blue P1, P2, P3, NB = navicular bone, PS = proximal sesamoid. The yellow ')' and '(' indicate where it is usually easiest to feel a 'digital pulse'.*

distribution of the arteries, veins and nerves prior to reaching the foot, but basic details should be helpful.

To a great extent the veins, arteries and nerves run down the leg in close proximity to each other, taking a route that provides them with protection, particularly from external trauma (damage). Two arterial branches travel down the leg, one to cover the lateral side (outside) of the leg and the second one the medial side (inside). They are protected by passing down the back of the leg, behind the knee and down the back (palmar surface) of the cannon bone, between the splint bones.

Different sections of the front (dorsal) part of the leg are supplied by individual branches from these two arteries as they pass down the back of the leg. When they reach the fetlock, if they continued down the palmar route over this joint, they would face being damaged by excessive and repeated stretching from dorsal flexion of the joint, so they take a route over the abaxial (outer) surface of the sesamoid bones, before returning to a more palmar position below this.

It is at this site, as the palmar arteries pass over the sesamoid bones, that it is easiest to palpate the 'digital pulse'; an increase in the strength of the digital pulse accompanies some foot conditions, such as an abscess or laminitis.

Foot Circulation

The blood vessels and nerves of the foot need to be protected from damage arising from the stretching and compression that occurs with every step that the horse takes, rather than from external injury, since they are protected by the hoof capsule. The larger arterial branches avoid direct compression by passing through the bone, or along grooves in its outer (dorsal) surface, and the circumflex artery of the sole runs around the foot beyond the perimeter of P3 rather than directly under it.

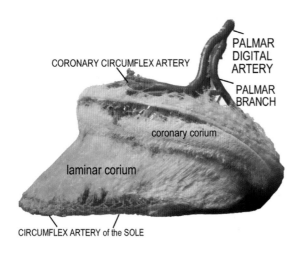

CORONARY CIRCUMFLEX ARTERY

PALMAR DIGITAL ARTERY

PALMAR BRANCH

coronary corium

laminar corium

CIRCUMFLEX ARTERY of the SOLE

Fig. 24   If latex is injected into the arteries of a cadaver specimen, and the other foot structures removed by acid treatment, a latex cast of the arteries and most of the capillary network can be produced.

To try to prevent damage from stretching, the blood supply to the laminae comes from a number of smaller arteries, mostly from branches of the terminal arch, each supplying a limited area of the laminae. A feature of the arterial supply to the foot is the way that different branches interconnect so as to, in effect, supply blood to the laminae from more than one direction, which helps to maintain perfusion of blood with the constant changes in pressure distribution.

The veins inside the hoof are unusual in that they do not have valves; thus the network of veins communicates more freely than in other tissues, and this allows the foot to compensate for uneven forces. I mentioned earlier how the hoof mechanism plays a part in returning blood to the heart by compression of the veins and the lymph vessels, and their position in the foot allows this. Concussive forces from foot loading are dissipated by this 'cushion' of fluid being forced out of these vessels when the foot lands.

Another feature of the foot circulation is the presence of arterio-venous (A-V) anastomoses, or 'shunts'. As well as the normal situation of blood passing from the arteries to the veins via the capillaries, these A-V shunts connect arterioles directly to venules. The discovery of

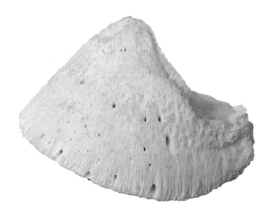

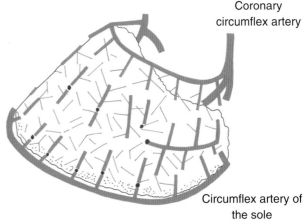

Coronary circumflex artery

Circumflex artery of the sole

Figs. 25a and 25b   The arterial blood supply to the laminae that cover the surface of P3. The lateral and medial digital arteries meet deep inside the structure of P3 at the terminal arch. Branches from the terminal arch exit through holes (foramen) in the bone. There are a number of foramina close to the distal border of P3, and the arterial branches that pass through these join together (anastomose) to form the circumflex artery of the sole (see Fig. 186).

these A-V shunts in the foot circulation led to the theory that blood was diverted through the shunts at the expense of capillary blood flow, and thus caused laminitis. However, it is far more likely that the A-V shunts have a thermo-regulatory role, as is the case when they are present in the tissues of other animals and birds. So when the A-V shunts are open, rather than diverting blood away from the capillaries, capillary flow is in fact maintained, and blood flows through both the shunts and the capillaries in order to warm the feet when they are too cold, and to cool them down when they are hot.

The Nerves of the Distal Limb

The medial and lateral palmer nerves (plantar nerves in the hind legs) accompany the vein and artery on each side of the leg. The nerves divide just above the fetlock to give dorsal branches that innervate (supply nerves to) the front (dorsal) part of the foot, and palmar branches that innervate the back of the foot (palmar).

The nerves in the foot are made up of vasomotor fibres to the blood vessels and sensory fibres from peripheral receptors that relay information to the spinal cord and brain. These messages may be of pain or heat, but also, by sending information about stretch and pressure, the body is able to sense the relative positions of the different structures of the foot, and thus the position of the foot on the ground and its relationship to the limb and body (proprioception).

THE INTEGUMENT: THE SKIN AND HOOF STRUCTURES

The integument refers to the outer layer of the body that covers and protects it. The majority of the integument is the skin, but it

also includes the hoof, frog and sole of the horse's foot. All these tissues are made up of two layers: an inner dermis, and an outer epidermis.

The Dermis

The dermis has a fibrous meshwork of collagen and elastin in which there is a variety of sensory nerve endings and a network of blood vessels, as well as adipocytes (fat cells), fibroblasts (that produce the collagen and elastin) and macrophages (protective cells, which destroy pathogens). Between the dermis and the epidermis that covers it, is a sheet of collagen, the basement membrane. If your skin is pinched, the strength of the collagen in the dermis and in the basement membrane prevents it from tearing, and when released the shape returns with the help of the elastin. You can see that blood is squeezed out by the pressure, with the skin going white, and the pain you feel is from one of a range of sensory receptors that are present in the dermis.

The dermis has large numbers of capillaries that provide nutrition for its own cells as well as for the epidermis outside it, which has no direct blood supply. Oxygen and nutrients spread from the capillaries into the dermis and pass through the basement membrane to reach the nearest epidermal cells. Because it is highly vascular (has many blood vessels), the dermis has an important role in body temperature control: thus when it is cold, the blood vessels are constricted (closed) to reduce blood flow and limit heat loss from the skin, and when it is hot they are dilated (opened), to try to lose heat and cool off.

Skin contains hair follicles and associated sweat and sebaceous glands in the dermis, which are also involved in the control of body temperature. Sweating is very important for a horse, as the evaporation of sweat helps prevent it from over-heating. In cold conditions, a horse

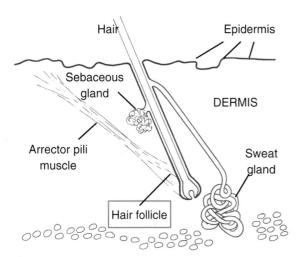

Subcutaneous tissue

Fig. 26   A hair follicle in the dermis of the skin. Contraction of the smooth muscle cells of the arrector pili muscle causes the hair to stand up. Sebaceous glands release sebum, an oily/waxy liquid, on to the hairs and skin surface to provide a protective waterproof cover.

can retain heat by making the hairs stand up, with the trapped air between the hairs acting as an insulating layer. Beneath the dermis of the skin is subcutaneous (under-skin) tissue, which has larger blood vessels that feed and drain the dermis and, as many of us are only too aware, is a site of storage for fat.

The Epidermis

The epidermis is the protective outer layer of the body that covers the dermis. As well as skin, epidermal tissues include nail, feather, hoof, hair and horn, and are characterized by the production of the fibrous protein, keratin; it is the presence of this protein in their cells which gives them the ability to provide protection to the underlying tissues. What happens to these cells (keratinocytes) – whether they are shed or retained – and also the type of keratin they contain, give the epidermal tissues their

different properties. Keratin can be divided into 'soft' keratin, found in skin, and 'hard' keratin as occurs in hoof. The hardness of keratin depends on the amount of the amino acid cysteine it contains, because cysteine's sulfur atoms are able to bind together to form strong bonds.

Under the microscope, there are several recognizable layers that make up the epidermis; these are identified as follows:

Stratum basale (basal cell layer): This is the innermost layer of cells, attached to the basement membrane. The basal cell layer is where cell division occurs, and as more cells are produced the older cells are pushed away from the dermis.

Stratum spinosum: As the cells move away from the dividing basal cells, they become filled with keratin fibres, and the nucleus and other internal cell structures degenerate and the cells die (keratinization).

Stratum granulosum: This layer is present in skin but absent in hoof tissues. Granules form in the keratinocytes and are released as the cells die, and this affects what happens to the outer layers of cells. In the skin, the release of the contents provides a protective waterproof covering to the cells, but also causes breakdown of the intercellular bonds that attach these cells to each other. This allows the superficial layers of dead skin cells to be shed (desquamate).

Stratum corneum: The outer layers of dead cells of the hoof structures, in the absence of the stratum granulosum, are not shed, and basal cell division pushes them down to the ground where they are worn away.

THE HOOF STRUCTURE

The hoof is a modified epidermal tissue, characterized by its hard keratin, the presence

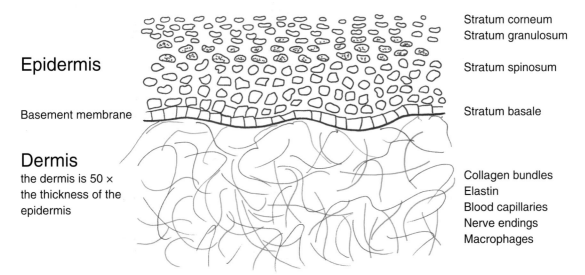

Epidermis

Basement membrane

Dermis
the dermis is 50 ×
the thickness of the
epidermis

Stratum corneum
Stratum granulosum

Stratum spinosum

Stratum basale

Collagen bundles
Elastin
Blood capillaries
Nerve endings
Macrophages

Fig. 27   The superficial layers of the skin.

of tubules in its structure, and the retention of the fully keratinized cells (rather than their being shed).

The Dermis

'Corium' is the term commonly used to refer to the dermis of the horny structures of the foot (*see* Fig. 17). The coronary corium provides nutrition for hoof production at the top of the wall, and the solar corium for the production of sole and frog corium for the frog, and they each have thin, cone-like projections (papillae) on their surface.

Again, under the microscope there are several recognizable growth layers that make up the epidermis, which are identified as follows:

Fig. 28   The black line depicts the layer of basal cells that divide to produce the hoof wall. The tubules are formed by the basal cells that line sockets into which the coronary papillae fit, and the inter-tubular horn is produced between them.

Stratum basale: The hoof, sole and frog grow by the division of basal cells, with those attached to a papilla forming a tubule and those in between the papillae dividing to produce intertubular horn. The inner surface

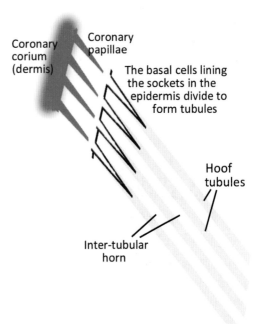

Coronary
corium
(dermis)

Coronary
papillae

The basal cells lining
the sockets in the
epidermis divide to
form tubules

Hoof
tubules

Inter-tubular
horn

of the hoof is joined to the laminar corium by the attachment of basal cells to its basement membrane. In normal circumstances these laminar basal cells divide slowly, contributing relatively little to overall hoof growth, but in response to injury they can multiply rapidly to repair any damage.

Stratum spinosum: As more layers of cells are laid down, keratinization takes place as the cells move through the stratum spinosum. For the intertubular horn, keratinization is complete by midway down the length of the dermal papillae. For tubular horn, the division of the basal cells lining the papillae produces rings of tubular horn, with keratinization occurring as the cells are pushed further away from the tubule basal cells.

Stratum corneum: The stratum corneum begins when the cells are fully keratinized and have died. Because of the angle of the coronary groove, this process is completed at a higher point on the outer wall than the inner wall, but even accounting for this, as well as the greater distance down the hoof wall for keratinization of the tubule cells, all cells will be keratinized within the top 2.5cm (1in) of the external hoof wall (*see* Fig. 29); therefore the stratum corneum includes most of the hoof wall.

'Stratum' is also the term used to refer to the different layers through the thickness of the hoof wall, namely the stratum externum, the stratum medium and the stratum lamellatum (or internum).

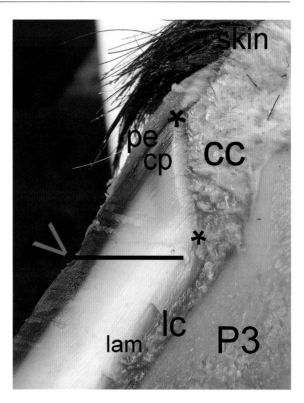

Fig. 29   The top of the dorsal hoof wall. The outer stratum medium in this foot has a thin strip of pigmented hoof outside unpigmented wall. The inner stratum medium and the stratum lamellatum are unpigmented. pe = the periople, lam = laminae (partially cut through in this section), lc = laminar corium, cp = coronary papillae, the pink strip of horn indicates how far the papillae extend down the wall (about 5mm), cc = coronary corium, and between the two '' is sometimes referred to as the 'coronary groove'.*
The red V (2.5cm – 1in – down the wall) shows the point on the external wall below which keratinization is complete even on the innermost part of the wall – at the end of the black line (approx. × 2 magnification).

The Stratum Externum/ Periople

The periople is the common name for the stratum externum, and is the thin layer of soft keratin that surrounds the top of the hoof wall. It encircles the hoof, including the heel bulbs where it blends with the frog, but rarely extends beyond a third of the way down the hoof wall, due to drying and being worn away. With its high lipid (fat) and moisture content, its role seems to be to reduce water loss from the growth layers at the top of the hoof wall, which helps to keep this area flexible.

The Stratum Medium

The stratum medium includes most of the thickness of the hoof wall. It is made up of tubular and intertubular horn, with different concentrations and types of tubule between its inner and outer zones. The tubules in the outer part of the wall are more concentrated, and the tubule shape changes from an oval shape near the outer wall to ones that are larger and rounder in the inner region.

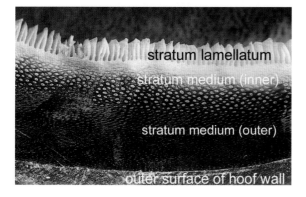

Fig. 30   The strata through the thickness of the hoof wall. The stratum lamellatum and inner part of the stratum medium are unpigmented, as are the tubule cells, seen in this picture as white dots in the inner stratum medium and white flecks in the outer stratum medium (the Type 3 tubules). The periople is absent from this section. (Image courtesy Dr Chris Pollitt)

Whether a hoof is black or not is governed by whether there are pigment-producing cells (melanocytes) in the basal cell layer where the new horn cells are formed, and this normally depends on whether there are melanocytes in the skin at the coronary band above it. Unpigmented (light-coloured) wall grows down below unpigmented (pink) skin, and pigmented horn below pigmented (black) skin. In dark feet, the amount of pigmented horn through the thickness of the wall is variable, and the intensity (darkness) of colour depends on the numbers of pigment cells present in the basal cell layer. Although sometimes suggested otherwise, the properties of unpigmented hoof appear to be no different from those of pigmented horn.

Even in pigmented hooves, the inner zone of the stratum medium and the stratum lamellatum are unpigmented, although small, localized areas of pigment occasionally occur in some feet. If the ground surface of the wall is rasped, this unpigmented strip of hoof horn can be seen just outside (abaxial to) what is referred to as the 'white line'.

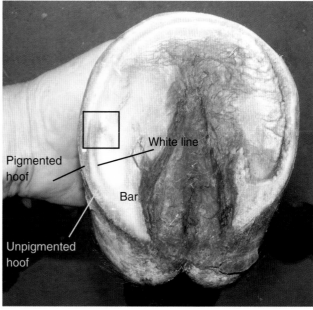

Fig. 31   Right fore of a Quarter horse. This shows how the unpigmented hoof ('zona alba') is lighter than the 'white line'. Pigment in the inner wall and 'white line' only ever seems to be in very localized areas (in box).

The Stratum Lamellatum (Internum)

The stratum lamellatum is the innermost part of the hoof wall, which has the leaves of horn that attach to the laminar corium. In books and articles, the terms 'laminae' and 'lamellae' are both used to refer to this junction. Microscopically, the leaves are made up of a thin layer of horn, commonly referred to as *primary epidermal lamellae*, and each one of these has multiple finger-like projections coming out from each side, known as the *secondary epidermal lamellae*. In this text I will refer to them as such, and will use 'laminae' to refer to the complete units, to include both the primary and secondary lamellae. These lamellae are attached to the dermis that fills the space between them, and are referred to as the *primary dermal lamellae* and the *secondary dermal lamellae* (*see* Figs 32 and 33). The primary epidermal lamellae originate from the inner edge of the coronary groove, and the basal cells keratinize as they move down and are fully formed by one third of the way down the hoof wall.

The Laminae

Hoof grows as the basal cells of the tubular and intertubular horn divide, pushing the older cells down till they eventually reach the ground. In order to be able to do this, the basal cells of the horny laminae have to be able to travel over the surface of the sensitive laminae (dermis) that is firmly attached to the surface of P3, while maintaining the overall strength of the hoof attachment.

Both the horny laminae and the sensitive laminae are bound to the basement membrane that lies between them. The strength of the junction is substantially increased by the large surface area provided by the secondary lamellae that branch out from the primary lamellae, this being a special feature of horses' feet.

To allow the hoof to grow down, Matrixmetallopropinase (MMP) enzymes, present in the dermis, break down the connection between basal cells of the secondary epidermal lamellae and the basement membrane. For the growing hoof, there must be an extremely precise balance between activation and inactivation of these MMP enzymes, allowing separation and re-attachment of the basal cells to let them move down (distally), and must occur in tiny areas at a time, so that the overall strength of the hoof attachment is not compromised.

Faint lines around the hoof, a few millimetres apart, indicate that there is a cyclical pattern to hoof growth, and these lines would appear to form from a brief cessation of growth between

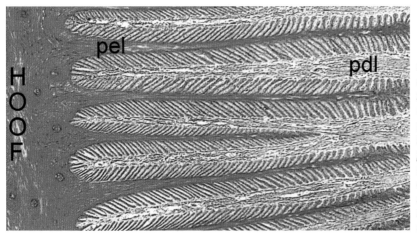

Fig. 32 *A transverse section across a hoof wall that is stained so that the collagen of the primary dermal lamellae (pdl) shows up blue and the keratin of the hoof and the primary epidermal lamellae (pel) is red. Each primary epidermal lamella has multiple secondary epidermal lamellae branching out from it. (Image courtesy Dr Chris Pollitt)*

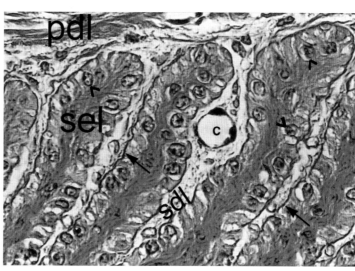

Fig. 33 Secondary epidermal and dermal lamellae stained to show keratin (red) and collagen (blue). The secondary epidermal lamellae (sel) are lined by basal cells, each one with its cell nucleus (arrow heads) and these are firmly attached to the sheet of collagen, the basement membrane that covers them (arrows). The tough connective tissue of the primary dermal lamella extends between the secondary epidermal lamellae, as secondary dermal lamellae (sdl), and is attached to the other side of the basement membrane. The dermis contains blood vessels and a capillary (c) can be seen between two secondary epidermal lamellae in this image. (Image courtesy Dr Chris Pollitt)

cycles. These 'growth rings' follow the shape of the coronary band and run parallel to it, and the spaces between the rings identifies the hoof growth occurring in each growth cycle. Hooves generally grow around 0.8cm ($^1/_3$ in) per month, with slower growth in winter than in summer. In cold conditions, blood vessels constrict to conserve heat, and the slower rate of growth is probably due to a combined effect of reduced blood flow and reduced enzyme activity at lower temperatures. In freezing conditions, the horse is able to maintain the temperature of its feet significantly lower than its core body temperature, and thus reduce heat loss from them and help conserve overall body heat. Intermittently the arterio-venous (A-V) shunts are opened, raising foot temperature and ensuring protection from freezing.

The Role of the Hoof Wall

The hoof wall has to be able to withstand impact forces from objects on its external surface as well as impact with the ground. It has to tolerate the more complex pattern of forces from the laminae, the ground reaction force, and consequent forces of deformation

of the hoof structure. It has to cope with the abrasion of its ground surface, and also deal with different environmental conditions – of wetness or dryness – as well as insulating the internal structures of the foot from extremes of temperature.

The forces acting on the hoof wall may be more fully identified as follows:

The forces from P3: Because of the very strong laminar attachment, when the foot takes weight, the forces from P3 are transferred to the surrounding hoof wall.

The ground reaction forces: These are the compressive forces on the hoof between the ground and the weight of the horse. They will depend on the speed the horse is travelling, the ground conditions and the weight of the horse (and rider). The percentage of a horse's weight carried by a fore foot is suggested as 0.3 (30 per cent) of the horse's weight when standing, increasing to the equivalent of 0.6 at the walk, 0.9–1.0 when trotting, and the equivalent of 1.75 times the weight of the horse at the gallop.

Forces of compression and tension in other directions occur due to changes in hoof shape resulting from the effects of weight and the opposing ground reaction forces.

The physical characteristics of the hoof (that enable it to deal with these forces):
Since it resembles an oblique cone, the overall shape of the hoof is relatively efficient at resisting bending, a cone being highly stable to bending in any axis. For the hoof this will be less effective when it is loaded unevenly – for instance if the horse has toe-in or toe-out conformation or if there is medio-lateral imbalance of the foot.

The strength of the hoof horn can partly be attributed to the amount and type of keratin in its cells, with the alignment of the keratin fibres appearing to be in the direction of the forces acting on the cell. The resilient fibre construction is the result of its strong disulfide bonds, and the characteristic smell of burnt hoof when a hot shoe is applied to the foot, is due to the burning of the sulfur in it (also the smell of sulfur from burnt hair).

The different distribution of the number and types of tubule through the thickness of the hoof gives the layers different properties. The higher concentration of tubules in the outer wall gives more protection to direct trauma to the hoof, and the oval shape of these tubules helps deal with the horizontal compressive forces from changes in hoof shape. It is the combination of tubular and intertubular horn that gives the hoof its strength and rigidity. The tubules act as supporting rods, but are reliant on the intertubular horn to support them and keep them straight.

The water content of the horn in the different layers affects their properties. The horn closest to the dermis contains the most water and the outer wall contains the least. The top inch of the hoof, that includes the stratum basale and stratum spinosum, has a high water content because it is close to the dermis, and it also has the periople to maintain hydration, so always remains flexible. The high moisture content of the laminae helps to give it the flexibility required to deal with the changing forces on this junction. The percentage of water in the laminae and inner wall is around 30 per cent, with a gradient down to 15–20 per cent in the outer layers. The water content of the outer wall will increase when the feet stand in mud and water, and hooves in these conditions are more flexible than when dry (similarly our nails are softer after we have taken a bath).

The Bars

If the hoof wall completely encircled the foot it would be far too rigid, but if it ended at the heels it would be too unstable – so the horse's foot evolved with a compromise, with the ends of the hoof wall turning inwards, to form the bars.

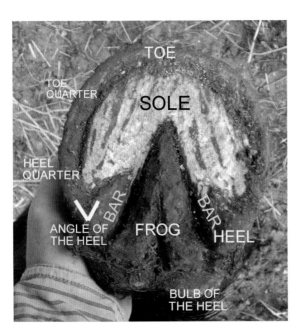

Fig. 34 The bars, on each side of the frog in the back half of the foot. The angle of the heel is the junction of the hoof and bar, 'V' in the picture.

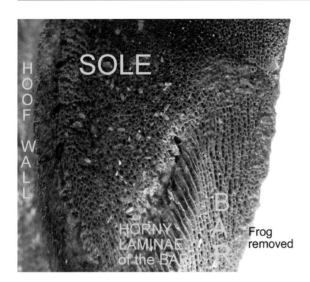

Fig. 35 The holes on the inner surface of this cadaver specimen are where the sole papillae of the solar corium would have fitted. The papillae of the bar corium would have fitted into the holes at the top of the bar. The bar grows down over the sensitive (dermal) laminae till it joins the sole and reaches the ground.

The bars start at the 'angle' of the heel, and run each side of the frog to about midway along its length. Their structure and growth are the same as for hoof horn, being produced from its corium and attached by laminae. The corium that produces the bar is connected to the hoof corium on its posterior (rear) border, to frog corium along its length, and to the sole corium on its anterior border.

The bars are important supporting structures of the foot, and are also involved with heel movement when the foot takes weight. Good 'foot function' does not just rely on individual healthy structures, but also on how they all work together and how the load is spread to the neighbouring tissues, and the bars have a role in this.

The Sole

The sole covers a large part of the bottom surface of the foot, and is formed by division of the basal cells attached to the solar corium. The cells keratinize and die as they move away from the corium, to produce the hard sole that we see when we pick up the foot. The surface of the solar corium is covered with short papillae, a few millimetres long, that produce tubular horn, and inter-tubular horn is formed between the tubules.

Rather than shedding the superficial dead cells, as skin does, or growing down as a unit like the hoof, the sole grows down in layers. This is most obvious in dried cadaver specimens (*see* Fig. 36), but is also evident in the way excess sole is shed in dry conditions. As a new layer is laid down, its tubular horn is embedded in the previous layer, resulting in a connection between the layers rather like the perforations in toilet paper. The water content of the internal layer of the sole is around 30 per cent, and changes little as the layers move away from the

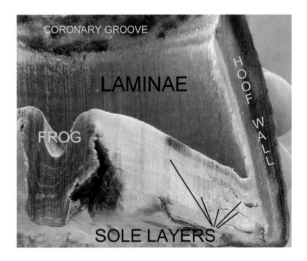

Fig. 36 With drying, the sole layers of this cadaver specimen have started to separate. In life, the deeper layers will remain moist and this drying will only happen to the superficial layer, allowing it to be shed. Separation between deeper layers can occur when pus uses the weak connection between the layers as an escape route for a sub-solar abscess (see Chapter 11). The light lines in the frog indicate that the frog also grows in layers.

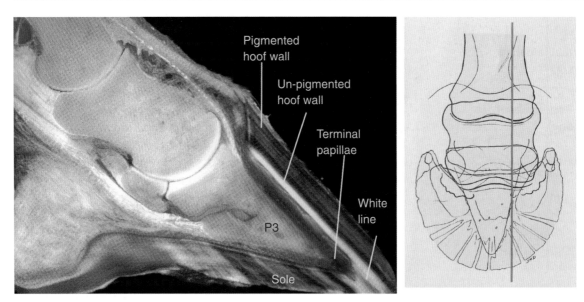

Fig. 37a *P3 is suspended from the hoof by the laminar attachment. The outer rim of the sole, stabilized by its attachment to the wall via the 'white line', helps to provide stability to the solar border of P3. (Image courtesy J-M. Denoix from* The Equine Distal Limb*)* **Fig 37b** *The line of the cut.*

dermis, until it becomes the most superficial layer. In dry conditions the superficial layer hardens as it loses moisture, and if it is not worn away through abrasion, develops cracks that allow areas of sole to break away. This ability to shed layers helps to prevent the sole from becoming too thick and inflexible. Growing in layers is also a safety mechanism, providing an escape route for pus from foot abscesses (*see* Chapter 11, Abscesses).

Although the sole has a role in helping to support the weight of the horse, it is not designed to bear weight and, other than perhaps the very perimeter of the sole, it should not make contact with the ground when the horse stands on a firm level surface. It helps to support the hoof wall by maintaining its shape, and we can see how distorted the over-grown hoof becomes once it has grown beyond the attachment to the sole. The sole will make contact with the ground if the horse is on a surface that allows the foot to sink into it, so has to be thick enough and strong enough to protect the internal structures of the foot

from damage or injury. Obviously a thicker sole provides a greater level of protection, but if it becomes too thick, from sole retention, it can limit the ability of the foot to flex and absorb concussive forces. This is sometimes referred to as being 'sole bound'.

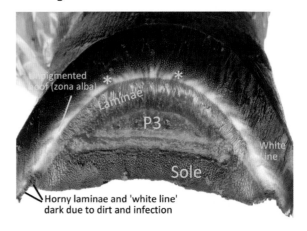

Fig. 38 *The lateral wall and sole of a pony's heavily pigmented foot. Pigment is included in the 'white line' and occasionally also extends into the 'unpigmented' stratum medium and stratum lamellatum (*) of the hoof wall.*

When weight is put on to a foot, the bone sinks relative to the hoof with stretching of its laminar attachments. The shape of the hoof means that these increased internal forces acting against the reactive ground forces tend to cause the hoof to expand, and a flexible sole allows it to do so. The sole follows the expansion of the wall, which causes it to flatten and lose its concavity, but by its firm attachment to it, it also limits the extent of the expansion. When exercising on soft ground, these forces of expansion are significantly reduced, and as the foot sinks into the surface, the space under the bottom of the foot is filled and the load is spread.

The White Line

The sole does not attach directly to the hoof wall but is connected to it by a narrow horny layer, the 'white line', which joins them firmly together and seals the gap between them. The sensitive laminae cannot extend beyond the limits of the dermal attachment to the bone, but the horny laminae continue down to the ground as the hoof grows, and if the dermal tissue did not change its form there would be a weak connection and poor seal between the hoof and the sole. At the distal end (bottom end) of the laminae, the dermal tissue changes to form 'terminal papillae' from which tubules are formed, and this, with surrounding intertubular horn, makes up the 'white line'.

The 'white line' is, in fact, a misnomer, since it is never white but usually a tan colour, and will be a blue/grey colour if the adjacent sole is pigmented. Confusion occurs because the strip of hoof on the inner edge of the hoof, adjacent to the 'white line', is always white, even in pigmented feet.

When the foot is picked up, in the shod foot the 'white line' is hidden by the shoe. In the unshod foot, the position of the 'white line' is identifiable often as a dirt line just inside

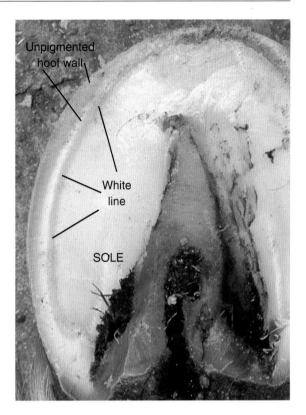

Fig. 39   This hoof is unpigmented, and externally will be a tan/yellowy colour. The outer wall is darker than the inner wall, which is white ('zona alba'). The 'white line' is the name given to the horn produced by the terminal papillae, and is the darker line between the hoof wall and the sole.

(axial to) any prominent hoof wall and outside (abaxial to) the smooth rim of the sole. In order to visualize the 'white line' and to identify its position and its relationship to the sole and the unpigmented hoof that it is attached to, the foot needs to be thoroughly cleaned and the embedded dirt in the bottom of the hoof wall rasped away.

The Frog

The frog is the wedge-shaped structure in the back half of the ground surface of the foot, lying between the bars and extending forward to a point in the central area of the sole; it is firmly attached to the digital cushion that lies above it (dorsal to it).

The high water content and its 'softer' keratin give the frog its rubbery form. The frog remains flexible provided it can maintain its moisture content, which the deeper layers, close to its corium, are able to do. In wet conditions even the superficial layer will remain pliable, but in dry environments the outer layer will dry out and can become extremely hard.

Like the sole, the frog grows down in closely attached layers (*see* Fig. 36). Sometimes whole layers of frog will be shed, however far more often only part of a layer will come away, and this leaves the frog with the ragged appearance that we generally see.

The frog gives protection to some important structures inside the foot. The deep digital flexor tendon, the coffin joint and the navicular bone and bursa lie directly above it, but only a very small part of the caudal (back) border of P3 (*see* Chapter 11).

Frogs can vary in shape and size, some being broad and voluminous, whereas others are thin and strap-like, and even though horses can remain perfectly sound with any shape or size of frog, a foot with a wider, more substantial one is likely to be more effective in providing traction and absorbing concussion. These broad frogs will often be accompanied by other foot structures that are also considered to be in their healthier and more functional form.

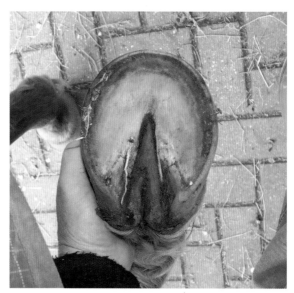

Fig. 41 Some frogs are thin and insubstantial.

IN CONCLUSION

We have seen how the foot is generally able to withstand the forces that act on it because all the structures in it play their part in absorbing or spreading the forces. In the following chapters it will be shown how the external features of the foot change when they fail to do so.

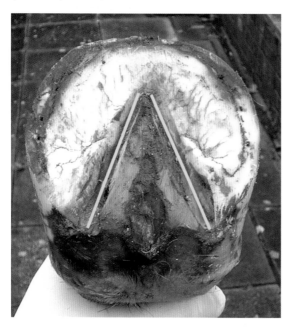

Fig. 40 The wedge-shaped frog is attached to the bars and sole at the depth of the collateral grooves (or collateral clefts) (yellow lines).

3 Examining the Feet

It is not difficult to identify a grossly misshapen foot, but experience is needed to work out what the deformity is, or to recognize a deformity in a foot where the changes are more subtle. Farriers and trimmers are able to identify stresses and imbalances from the foot shape and the wear of the shoe or hoof, but even for them, working out how to correct them can be a challenge. The good news is that every horse or pony has four feet which can be studied if you wish to gain experience.

The examination of a horse's feet does not just involve picking them up and looking at them, but includes observing the horse's conformation and demeanour from a distance to see how it stands and moves. Regarding its conformation, the following points might be considered:

- Do the legs appear to be in proportion to the body (are they too long or too short)?
- Are the different parts of the leg in proportion?
- Are the legs straight?
- Do they appear rotated?
- Are the feet turned in or out?

Then take a note of the horse's stance:

- How are the legs positioned? Does the horse stand square, or are the feet set under the body?
- Is the hoof-pastern axis straight?
- Does the horse stand with one foot set forward or back?

Feet will be assessed by the farrier or trimmer at their routine visits, but very often owners will not really look at them unless they have noticed an obvious defect, or if the farrier points out some change in them.

There are some people – and I hope you are now one of these – who like to study horses' feet to try to understand how they function and how they become distorted, but otherwise, probably the two most common situations for feet to be examined closely are when a horse is looked at prior to purchase, and when a horse is lame. I will therefore use these two scenarios as the basis of an examination: first, when you do not know the horse and are looking at it with an interest in buying it; and second, when your horse, which you know well, goes lame.

THE PRE-PURCHASE EXAMINATION

To properly assess conformation and stance, a horse should be standing square on a flat level surface, ideally with the front and hind feet lined up together, and it should be examined from all sides. Unfortunately, finding a flat surface for the horse to stand on can be difficult, and getting a horse to stand completely square is often impossible.

'Conformation' describes the horse's structural form, and 'stance' its posture. Regarding conformation, the body and limb proportion – which will vary according to

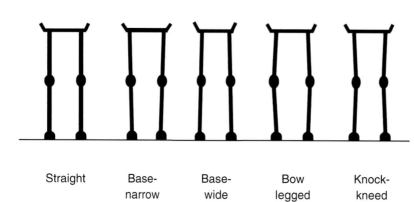

Fig. 42 Different forelimb conformations.

| Straight | Base-narrow | Base-wide | Bow legged | Knock-kneed |

breed – needs to be considered, as well as the alignment of the limbs in relation to the body, and the feet relative to the limbs. An 'ideal' conformation is one where all limb structures are loaded evenly, in all four legs, but this is probably rarely found. Judgement of conformation has to be based on whether a particular feature is more likely to load any part of the limb abnormally, thus making it more liable to damage and to cause lameness.

The horse should be examined from in front and from behind, and considered in the light of the following conformational faults:

- The legs are not perpendicular when seen from in front or from behind: this might be **'base narrow'**, where the feet are closer together than the top of the leg; or **'base wide'**, where the feet are wider apart than the top of the leg.
- The axis of all or part of the limb is rotated: this might be **'toe in'** (pigeon-toed), where the toes point inwards; or **'toe out'** (splay-footed), where the toes are turned outwards.
- The angulation of specific joints is changed: this might be in the knee, where the knees are either outside the mid-line – known as **bow legged** – or closer together, known as **knock kneed**; or it might be in the hocks,

where the hocks are either outside the mid-line – known as **bow legged** – or closer together, known as **cow hocked**.

There is obviously a close correlation between conformation and stance, but there are several reasons why a horse's stance might change while its conformation remains unchanged. Most commonly this will be from changes in the way the feet are trimmed or shod, but also the limb position may be altered due to pain.

There are certain features that can be attributed solely to structural differences, including rotation of the axis of the leg, causing the feet to turn in or out, and misalignment of joints – but sometimes it can be difficult to work out how much a horse's limb position is the result of its conformation, or how much is due to the shape of the foot.

Certain conformational features commonly occur together, with 'toe in' often accompanying 'base narrow', and 'toe out' often accompanying 'base wide'. For horses with a 'base narrow' conformation, the outside of the leg (the lateral side) will be subjected to greater forces and will consequently be more liable to injury, whereas in those that are base wide the inside of the leg (the medial side) is more likely to be affected. For individual joints that are not in the median plane, such as bow legs, the collateral ligaments will be more stressed on the stretched side, and it will be the bones on the medial side that are more likely to suffer damage.

When it comes to examining the feet, evidence of these uneven forces may be apparent from changes in the hoof. Due to its conformation, a horse's action may load the foot unevenly and cause a change in foot shape – but equally, changing the trim or shoe can alter the way a horse stands and moves. This is why it is important to examine the horse's conformation, stance and movement, as well as the feet, to try to work out which it is.

Changes in Stance

Horses will very rarely be seen standing completely square with both front and hind feet in alignment, as the four legs on a table. The front legs will be seen aligned far more commonly than the hinds, because of the way that horses intermittently rest the hind legs. A 'normal' stance is generally said to be when a horse stands square with the elbow to the fetlock in the front legs, and the hock to the fetlock in the hind legs, perpendicular to the ground, with the change in angle at the fetlock

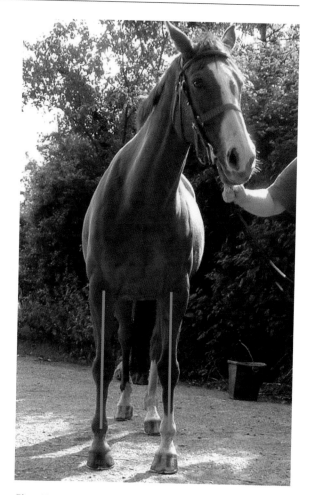

Fig. 43   Toe-in conformation.

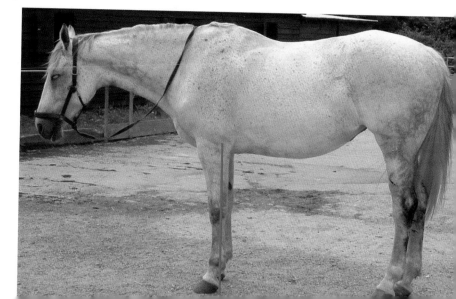

Fig. 44   Standing almost completely 'square' (on all four legs), close to what is suggested to be a 'normal' stance.

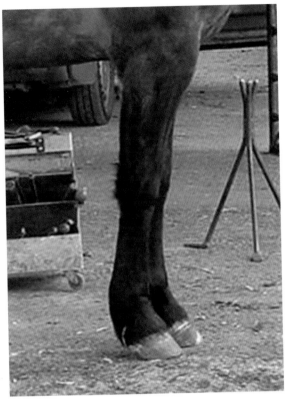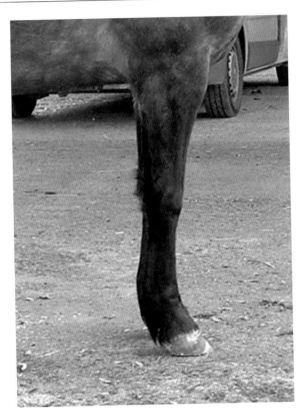

Figs. 45a and 45b   Prior to trimming, this pony was 'standing under' on both front legs. Its stance changed after the left fore was trimmed (left), and after the right fore was done, stood square on them both (right).

so that if a plumb line were hung from the lateral epicondyle (on the outside) of the elbow, it would line up with the bulbs of the heel. The other feature considered important is a straight alignment of the pastern and the dorsal hoof wall.

In other literature, horses with fore limbs angled back under the body (known as 'standing under'), or held extended forwards (known as 'camped'), are often described as having a 'conformational abnormality'. Likewise, the hind leg position when it angles forwards under the body or extends backwards – again known as 'standing under' and 'camped behind' – is also considered to be abnormal. This is very often not the case. Certainly the forearm and cannon need to be aligned to remain stable when the horse

stands or moves, and likewise the alignment of the phalanges needs to be straight (a straight hoof-pastern axis); however, the positioning of the leg and the angle of the pastern depend, to a great extent, on how the feet are trimmed.

The Hoof-Pastern Axis (HPA)

The hoof-pastern axis (HPA) refers to the line of the hoof and pastern when looked at from the side, and is used as an indication of the alignment of the phalangeal bones. In order to maintain even forces when the horse stands or moves, the HPA should be straight – where the front (dorsal surface) of the pastern and the dorsal hoof wall are at the same angle. A horse can have a straight HPA with a range of different hoof angles, and it achieves this by changing its stance. This adaptability does not fit with the 'normal' stance described previously, but is demonstrated in the example in Fig. 45. In this case, the pony has a straight HPA both before and after trimming, and what has changed is its leg position. The concept that horses can have a straight HPA without having a perpendicular limb seems to be universally ignored, and in many books and articles, photographic examples of how a foot has been trimmed to produce a straight HPA pays no attention to the different position of the limb in the 'before' and 'after' pictures.

The use of 'normal stance' (perpendicular limb and straight HPA) applies to only a limited range of hoof angles, and it is not how horses with upright feet usually stand. This might be understandable if these higher hoof angles were considered abnormal, but they are not. The range of front hoof angles which has been suggested as being normal is between 45 and 60 degrees. For the most part, horses with angles within this range are able to maintain a straight HPA by changing the angle of the limb. Beyond these limits, the hoof will be more upright than the pastern – 'broken forward' – or will have a lower angle than the pastern –

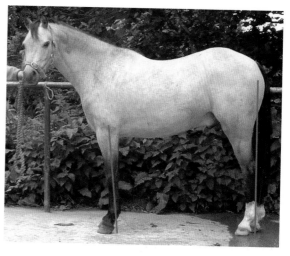

Fig. 46   Pony with hoof angle over 55 degrees, 'standing under' with a straight hoof-pastern axis. Perpendicular hind limb position.

'broken back' – both of which are more likely to lead to problems. (If the limb is actually positioned with the leg vertical, as is often done by vets when taking radiographs, this 'unnatural' position for many upright feet will inevitably give them the appearance of having a 'broken forward' HPA.)

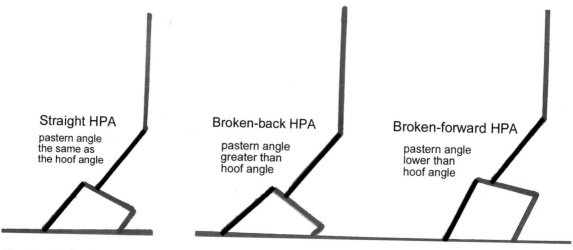

Straight HPA
pastern angle the same as the hoof angle

Broken-back HPA
pastern angle greater than hoof angle

Broken-forward HPA
pastern angle lower than hoof angle

Fig. 47   The hoof-pastern axis.

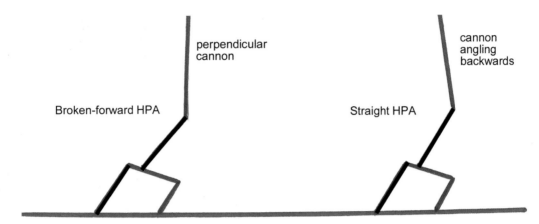

Fig. 48   If an upright foot is positioned with a perpendicular cannon, the HPA would be broken-forward (left) but horses with feet at this angle will generally alter their stance and maintain a straight HPA (right).

The Horse's Action

Having observed the horse standing, it should be seen walking and trotting on a firm, level surface. This gives the opportunity to see how any conformational issues affect the way the horse moves. The relevance of poor conformation is that the horse will often have an action that is not straight, and the feet may land nearer the midline (plaiting), or away from it when the foot may swing in (winging) or out (paddling), and result in unbalanced forces on the feet on landing – for example, base-narrow horses generally land on the lateral wall.

Other things to observe include the following:

● Is the stride length the same for both front legs, and also for the hind pair?
● How do the feet land? When the horse

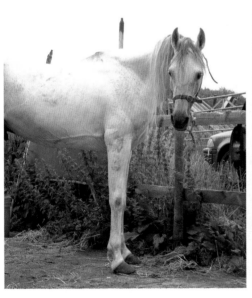

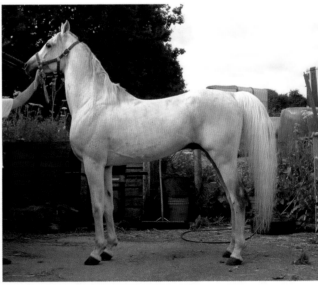

Figs. 49a and 49b   LEFT: An Arabian stallion with a severely broken back HPA after the farrier was eight weeks late for his routine ten week appointment! RIGHT: Five days later after the farrier had been, with a 'normal' stance and straighter HPA.

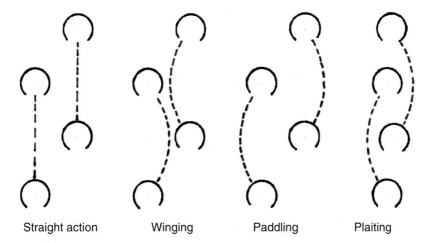

| Straight action | Winging | Paddling | Plaiting |

Fig. 50 Different fore limb actions.

walks, do the feet land flat, or with the toe hitting the ground first, or do they land obviously heel first?

● When seen from in front and behind, do the feet land evenly, or do they land obviously on the outside or inside wall, and is it the same at walk and at trot?

Assessment of the Feet

Before each individual foot is examined closely, try to judge whether the feet are in proportion to the rest of the body, and also whether they are a matching pair both in front and behind.

Feet that seem to be too large for the rest of the body generally are so because they are overgrown, particularly if they have been allowed to spread, and their proportion will be improved by a good trim.

If a horse's feet are small relative to its body size, the force per area on them is greater and they may not be able to withstand the forces they are subjected to. This will depend, to some extent, on what the horse is wanted for – a lighter workload, a lighter rider and leaner condition of the horse all improve the chances of these horses staying sound.

Mis-matched Feet

There is often some difference between the left and right feet of a horse, but in most cases this will not be obvious. It is the front feet that are far more commonly 'mis-matched', with one foot more upright and 'boxy', and the other one lower and more spread (*see* High/Low Feet, Chapter 4).

A number of things need to be considered if you are contemplating buying a horse with this conformation:

● How great is the disparity between the feet?
● Is one foot too upright or the other foot too low, or are both 'abnormal'?
● How do they affect the horse's stance and action?

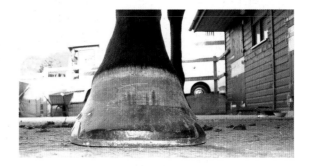

Fig. 51 Thoroughbred × Warmblood with an overgrown splayed foot.

- How old is the horse? Beyond the age of four, the horse can be considered 'fully developed', and the likelihood of being able to 'correct' the situation will be limited.
- What is the intended use of the horse – the speed and intensity of the work, the weight of the rider, and so on?

Having markedly different feet must inevitably cause some imbalance to the rest of the body, and although a horse with high/low front feet can remain sound throughout its life, the more it is required to do and the greater the difference between the feet, the more likely it will be for such a case to develop problems.

The Shod Horse

If the horse is shod the shoe will limit examination of the parts of the foot that lie under it. The type of shoe can be checked,

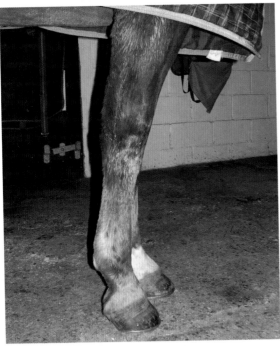

Fig. 52 An Irish Draught with an upright right fore and left fore with a lower hoof angle. Different limb positions, both with a straight HPA – see Chapter 5.

however, and the vendor may be able to explain why a certain type of shoe has been used, if it is different from the normal plain shoe. A particular shoe may just be the choice of the farrier, but it may have been applied to counteract some deformity, or to change the mechanics of the foot to improve its action, or in response to lameness.

The placement and fit of the shoe needs to be checked. Is it fitted to the entire rim of the foot, and does the edge of the shoe lie outside the hoof wall, or does the edge of the wall overlap the shoe? How far back do the branches of the shoe go: are they to the back of the heels, or do they stop short of them, or extend beyond them? The position of the nail clenches can be checked, and whether they still lie tightly to the outside wall. Because the relative position of some of these features will change in the period between shoeings, you need to know when the horse was last shod.

Most working horses in the UK are shod, and if you intend to carry on in the same way, seeing how it is shod will be relevant. However, it will be more difficult to tell how the horse might cope with going barefoot, if that is your intention.

Close Examination of the Feet

A close examination of the feet will reveal obvious defects such as splits or cracks; other, less obvious changes are listed below. The relevance of all these changes will be covered in later chapters.

From in front:

- Are the hoof tubules straight? Do the middle tubules of the dorsal wall end up centrally at the toe, or are they angled to one side?
- Are the medial and lateral sides of the hoof at obviously different angles? (It is normal for the medial wall to be very slightly more upright than the lateral wall.)

- Is there any flaring of the walls?
- Is the coronary band level across the front of the foot, or higher on one side?

These features are useful indicators of medio-lateral balance or imbalance.

From the side:

- Is there any change in the line of the dorsal wall, or is it straight?
- Are the growth rings even around the foot, or do they diverge and become wider apart at the heels?
- Are the tubules around the hoof at the same angle as those of the dorsal wall, or do they progressively become lower towards the heel?
- Is the coronary band on the side of the foot in a straight line, or is it curved?

The solar surface:

- Is there an obvious difference between the lateral and medial halves of the foot?
- Does the sole have concavity, or does it appear flat?
- Are there raised areas of the sole, or is it smooth and even?
- Is the frog narrow or is it wide, and is its surface smooth, or ragged and pitted?
- Is there a good connection between the wall and sole, or does it appear crumbly or wider than it should be?
- Are the bars straight, or are they curved and flattened?
- Are the heels collapsed? Is the heel horn turned under and growing forward to cover the sole?

EXAMINING THE LAME HORSE

All the same features have to be considered when looking for possible foot lameness as when looking at a prospective purchase. The difference is that, when the horse is your own, its conformation and normal stance will be known to you, and what you will be looking for is any difference in these, and any physical changes in one leg compared to the opposite, sound leg. Ask someone to walk and trot the horse for you so that you can see it move.

Working out which leg a horse is lame on is not always that easy, particularly if it is only slight and there is no evidence of any injury or swelling visible anywhere. The lameness may well be accompanied by nodding of the head, but some owners are confused by this, as demonstrated by the number of times I have been asked to look at a horse that is lame on a particular leg, and it turns out to be the opposite one. The way a horse moves will differ depending on which part is affected, but for a foot problem, it will invariably be more painful at some point in the stance phase when weight is on the affected leg. This is accompanied by lifting of the head, as the horse attempts to manoeuvre the body to reduce loading the painful foot, followed by dipping of the head when weight is transferred on to the opposite sound leg.

Some confusion can occur if a horse has pain moving a front leg, such as, for example, with a muscle strain, since this coincides with the other limb taking weight. Trotting the horse in a circle may help to differentiate between the two, and assessing the degree of lameness on different surfaces can also be helpful. Painful conditions of the foot generally are worse on hard surfaces, whereas a 'moving-leg lameness' is less likely to change.

Head bobbing can also occur when lameness comes from a hind leg, and again there can be confusion because at trot, the diagonal feet are on the ground at the same time, so a right hind foot lameness can be mistaken for lameness on the left fore. Generally, movement of the head is less obvious and less consistent when a horse is lame on a hind leg, and can usually be differentiated by more obvious movement of the hindquarters and changes in stride length, which again may be more evident in a circle.

Foot placement may change, depending on the site of pain in the foot, taking a shorter stride when the pain is in the back of the (palmar) foot and placing the foot further forward when there is toe pain, or placed abaxially (away from the body) if the pain is in the lateral part of the foot. If the lameness is mild, there may be no change in stance, but a foot positioned just slightly ahead of the other could possibly indicate navicular disease, while one resting on the toe is likely to indicate heel pain.

The palmar digital artery passes over the outside of the sesamoid bones, and it is at this site that a 'digital pulse' is palpable. The strength of this pulse is increased particularly in laminitis, but also with inflammatory processes going on in the foot, with abscesses or with bruising. Feeling a pulse takes a bit of experience, but it is well worth taking the time to practise locating it, because the presence of a strong digital pulse is diagnostic of a problem involving the foot (*see* Figs 23 and 130).

Practical Aids for Foot Assessment

Some simple pieces of equipment can help identify imbalance and abnormalities when starting to study feet, or when assessing a foot before trimming, the simplest being a ruler and a marker pen. Thus a line drawn down the central tubules of the dorsal wall can show whether they are straight or angled to one side, which can help to identify medio-lateral imbalance. With the foot lifted, a line can be drawn from the central cleft of the frog through its point (apex) and extended to the toe, which can demonstrate whether there is a marked difference between the medial and lateral sides of the foot.

A line drawn across the widest part of the foot can demonstrate how much of the ground surface is in front of this line and how much behind it.

Some relatively simple and inexpensive instruments are available, which while they are promoted primarily as aids to trimming and foot preparation, can also be helpful when assessing feet. A **'T'-square** can help identify the alignment of the foot in relation to the limb,

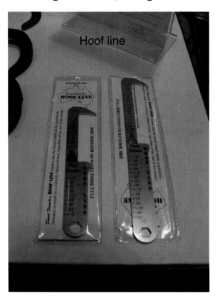

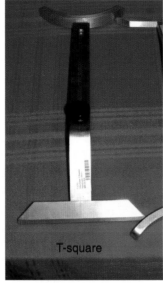

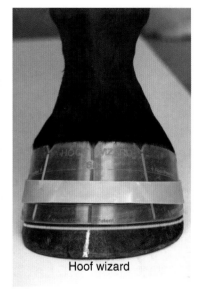

Figs. 53a, 53b and 53c Instruments marketed as aids for trimming, but they can also be useful for assessing feet.

and can also show the balance of a trim. **Hoof gauges** can be used to measure hoof angles – except that they measure a part of the wall that is often deformed, so are probably of limited benefit.

Medio-lateral imbalance is made more obvious by the use of a '**Hoof Wizard'**, which can help demonstrate imbalance relative to the midline. Similarly hoof boots whose front edge is below the level of the coronary band can be used to show imbalance relative to the ground surface (the trim), by drawing a line to mark the top edge of the boot.

Finally the **PAD** is a piece of perspex (Plexiglas) with lines marked on it, making angles. This is based on the template for trimming used by Strasser trimmers, but can be extremely useful for assessing horses' feet. How I used this in my investigation of feet, and the conclusions I have come to, are dealt with in detail in the final chapter.

Photographing Feet

Photographs can easily be taken with digital cameras, and these have a big advantage over SLR cameras because unsatisfactory pictures can be seen at the time, deleted, and new ones taken. They also have the advantage that computer software allows manipulation to improve the final image.

A good set of photographs records the shape and condition of the foot at that particular point in time, and has the following further advantages.

- They allow you to study the form of the foot at your leisure. This may help you to identify hoof imbalances and deformities.
- They can be used to monitor changes occurring in the feet, or to record the progress of remedial (corrective) work.
- They can be sent to other people to get further opinions about the state of the feet.

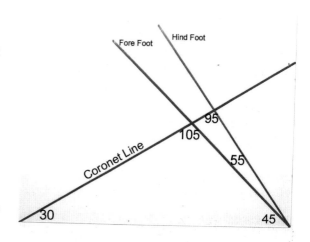

Fig. 54   The 'PAD' (see Chapter 12).

- If you are interested in buying a horse some distance away from where you live, you can send them to your vet and farrier so they can give their opinion on any apparent deformity, since it is they who will be involved with the horse's care.
- Photographs can be taken at the same time, and from the same position, as radiographs, so they can be compared.

The Importance of Photographic Technique

First of all, you must be able to see the entire foot. All those photographs of beautiful Thoroughbred stallions standing in grass are probably not taken there just for aesthetic reasons, but to hide their feet. Even standing the horse on dirt will hide the bottom edge and will often not be completely level. *Stand the horse on a level area of concrete.*

Do not take photographs too close to the subject (a macro setting on the camera may allow close-up images to be taken). Clear away objects in the foreground that an automatic focus might react to. *The foot must be in focus in the image.*

It can be difficult to identify things if the

image is too dark, or if there are areas of light and shade. Using the camera flash will help to provide a bright and evenly lit image, but reflection may be a problem if the feet are wet. For everyone's safety, try the flash away from the horse first, to ensure that it will not be frightened by it. *Adequate lighting is required.*

The hoof wall should be cleaned to remove dirt so that growth rings and tubule alignment can be assessed. Hair from the pastern and coronet (feathers) should be held, or taped up,

out of the way so that the top of the hoof wall can be seen. The solar surface of the foot needs to be picked out and thoroughly cleaned. *Good foot preparation is important.*

Although setting the camera on the highest pixel level provides the best picture and allows greater versatility for any alteration on the computer, it can be a disadvantage when trying to send images over the internet. *Take photographs with the appropriate pixel setting for your requirements.*

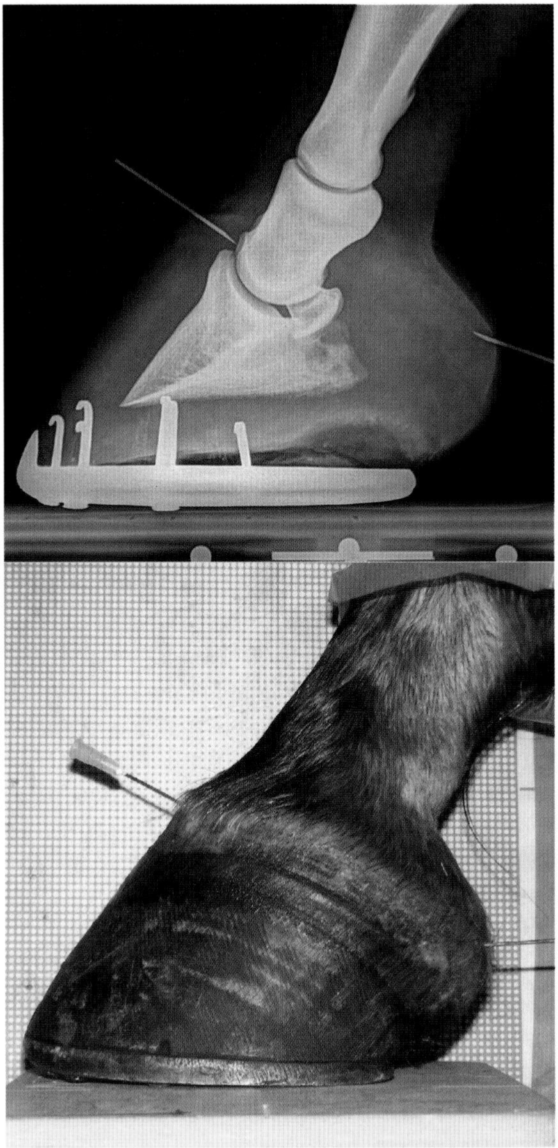

The Importance of Positioning

Photographs taken from a standing or kneeling position, as so often appear in articles and books, may identify a deformity but often will tell you very little more than this. Photographs taken at ground level will give far more information.

Positioning of the camera relative to the foot will depend on whether there is a particular feature that you want to record, but regardless of what other directions you take photographs from, some should always be taken from ground level directly in front of the foot and directly from the side (the lateral aspect). Photographs taken from ground level will allow you to see tubule alignment, deviation of the wall, and any variation in the growth rings, which are more likely to indicate the cause of any deformity. Note that it is not necessary for the photographer to lie down on the ground to line up the photograph: taking the pictures with the camera placed on, or close to, the ground is usually satisfactory.

There are other views of the foot that can be useful when assessing its form and balance. The medial view – the inside hoof wall – can be taken and compared with the lateral view, though the opposite leg will probably need to

Fig. 55 A photograph and a radiograph can be taken for comparison (cadaver specimen).

be lifted. Also useful is the view of the heels with the foot on the ground, though due to personal safety precautions, this shot can be difficult to line up correctly.

More photographs can usefully be taken with the foot lifted up (be sure that it is picked out and cleaned). Firstly a solar view can be taken, which is at right angles to the bottom of the foot, to assess the ground surface of the foot. Also a picture of the heels may be useful, taken at the back of the foot, to view the heel alignment and balance; and finally a half-solar view, taken from the back of the foot with the sole at an angle, to judge the in-turn of the heels and the curvature of the bars.

If specific measurements are required from the photographs, it will help to attach visible markers to the foot; combining this with more specific positioning of the camera will give the most accurate results. Including an object of known length or a scale ruler in the photograph will enable true measurement of length and distance to be calculated. Applying markers to the hair-line of the coronary band at the top of the dorsal wall and at the bulb of the heel will make it easier to measure the dorsal wall and heel to ground angles, and also that between the dorsal wall and the line of the coronet.

The truest results will be obtained if the camera is aligned at the level of, and at right angles to, the angle being measured, but this may be difficult to line up, and an image

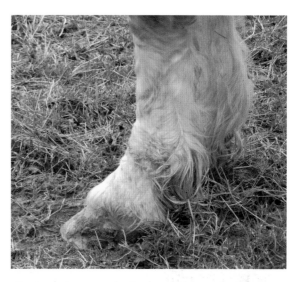

Fig. 56 Photograph of a pony's foot with the pony stood in a field, with hair and mud covering the foot and taken from a poor position. This photo is useless for assessment purposes!

taken aimed at the centre of the foot is usually adequate.

IN CONCLUSION

So the feet have been closely examined; obvious defects such as splits or cracks have been noted, and other, less obvious changes have been listed. The relevance of all of these changes will be covered in later chapters.

4 The Hoof

A hoof that is evenly loaded and functioning efficiently has the following features: a straight wall with no folds or flares, tubules running parallel and even growth rings around the foot, a heel angle close to the dorsal (front) wall angle, the medial half of the foot very similar to the lateral side, concavity of the sole, and a broad frog that makes contact with the ground when the foot takes weight. These features not only indicate that the foot structures are all working well together, but also that the horse has a good conformation and good action, both of which load the foot evenly. Any factor that disadvantageously affects the even loading of the foot or the functional dynamics of the internal foot structures will, over time, lead to changes in the hoof wall.

Hooves come in many shapes and sizes without apparently being deformed, but are they all normal? This chapter will investigate the factors affecting hoof shape, from the strength

of the hoof wall, hoof angle and hoof growth, to the way the foot is trimmed and balanced.

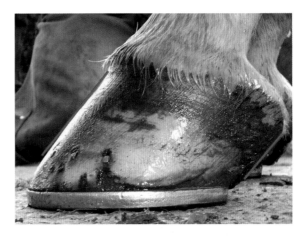

Fig. 58   A strong foot with the heel angle the same as the dorsal wall (the left fore of a Lusitano).

THE STRENGTH OF THE HOOF WALL

When I had taken photographs of the feet of over a thousand horses and ponies, I thought I might be able to categorize the foot type of the different breeds – but I found I was unable to do so because there were too few examples of many breeds and too many cross-breds. Nevertheless I soon realized that there was a pattern to the shape of the hooves and the way they deformed in response to uneven forces, and that this seemed to correlate with the

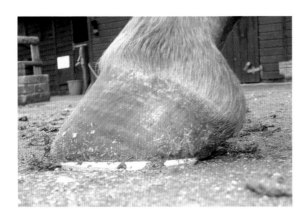

Fig. 57   A 'normal' foot (shod).

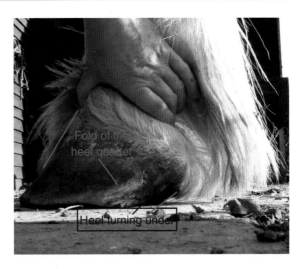

strength of the hoof wall relative to the weight of the horse.

Some breeds, such as the Andalusian and Arabian, have strong walls which retain their shape and only deform when the foot is very overgrown, while at the other end of the spectrum are breeds with weak-walled feet, most typically the Thoroughbred. If strong feet are allowed to grow long, they tend to grow down in a more cylindrical shape, and the heel angle remains similar to the dorsal wall angle, whereas weak feet easily deform under load, typically with flaring of the wall, heels folding under and flattening of the sole. A similar pattern of deformation can be seen in the feet of some other breeds, for example the Clydesdale, and although obviously stronger than the feet of the average Thoroughbred, their hooves are sometimes not strong enough to cope with their greater weight.

Most horses have strength of hoof somewhere in between the two extremes, and the characteristics of deformation in response to loading will be closer to one or other, depending on how strong or weak they are. Strong hooves are able to maintain a higher hoof angle because their heels are capable of staying upright. The heels of feet with weaker hooves always turn inward to some degree, and this results in a difference between the dorsal wall and heel angles, as well as some loss of heel height.

Hoof thickness must play a part in hoof strength, but differences in the number and distribution of laminae around the foot, or tubule distribution through the wall, may also be involved. Differences in hoof wall thickness are evident on radiographs: for instance, that of heavy horses with larger feet can measure over

20mm from the outer hoof wall to the bone, whereas it may be only 15mm in thoroughbreds – though this does also include the thickness of the dermis. The hoof wall at the heels is thinner and more flexible than the dorsal wall, but the concentration of laminae (the number of laminae per centimetre) is also less at the heels, and this presumably also affects flexibility. The total number of laminae in a foot (generally 500–600) appears to vary between breeds, and

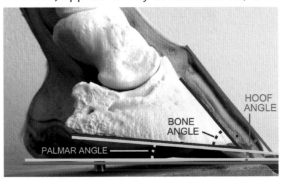

Fig. 60 Hoof Angle = the angle of the dorsal hoof wall to the ground = the angle the top inch of the dorsal wall makes with the horizontal.

P3 Bone Angle = the angle the dorsal surface of P3 makes with its solar border.

Palmar Angle = the angle of the solar border to the ground = the angle the line joining the lowest points of the solar border makes with the horizontal.

this must affect the strength and rigidity of the hoof structure.

HOOF ANGLES

The 'hoof angle' is the angle between the dorsal hoof wall and the ground-bearing surface

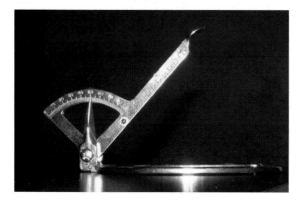

Fig. 61   A hoof gauge.

of the wall, or the ground if the foot is on a hard, flat surface. The debate about what a 'correct' hoof angle should be has been going on for centuries, with a range of suggestions anywhere between 45 and 60 degrees. There are a number of models of hoof gauge that have been produced to measure the hoof angle, but because they generally measure the lower half of the hoof wall, which is often deformed, they turn out to be not particularly accurate and have been shown to produce inconsistent results in the hands of different operators, so their use is somewhat limited. For the individual user, the results are likely to be more consistent, and some farriers and trimmers do use hoof gauges to monitor hoof angles in their work, but it is not common practice.

Although suggested numbers for hoof angles are still often given, farriers and trimmers more commonly use a straight hoof-pastern axis (HPA) as an indicator as to how a foot should

be trimmed. The bones of the digit must act as a unit as the horse moves, to be able to absorb forces efficiently without stressing any particular part. If not straight, the joints would be liable to hyperextension or flexion and collapse, which would be more likely to result in injury.

Using the HPA, a 45-degree hoof angle turns out to be too low because many of these have a broken back HPA, and those with around a 60-degree hoof angle are generally broken forward. In between these angles, a horse is usually able to compensate by altering its stance to maintain a straight HPA, so if just relying on

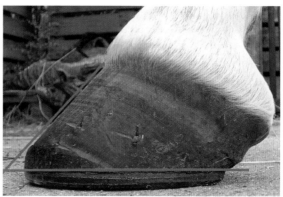

Fig. 62   The strong hoof of an Arab trimmed to about 47 degrees. Hooves at this angle are far more commonly found in weaker feet with collapsed heels.

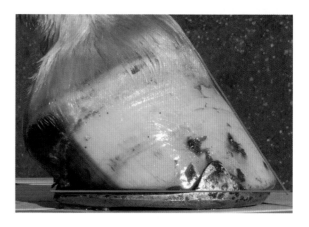

Fig. 63   A forefoot with hoof angle of around 57 degrees.

this as an indicator for a 'correct' angle, any suggestion for a hoof angle between 47 and 57 degrees could be considered as 'normal'. Actually, all this tells us is that a horse with front feet within this range of angles is more likely to stay sound than one that is outside this range – but it is not necessarily the best angle for the horse.

BONE POSITION IN THE FOOT

So what is the bone position in the feet with these variations in hoof angles? In feet that have intact laminae, the shape of the hoof reflects the shape of P3, so one possibility would be that the bone shape is different in feet with these different angles – and at first glance, it does appear that cadaver specimens of P3 do come in a great variety of shapes (and sizes). In the same way that hooves deform as the result of constant stress, so does the form of P3 adapt and remodel over time, and this, to some extent, accounts for the variation in bone shape. However, if we concentrate on the area around the centre of the bone where there is the least distortion, and ignore the periphery, a far greater consistency appears – and this is of a bone with a dorsal angle of close to 45 degrees (*see* Chapter 12). With a reasonable consistency of P3 bone angle, and provided there is good laminar attachment, a foot with a higher hoof angle will contain a bone with a greater palmar angle (the angle of the solar border to the ground) than one with a lower hoof angle.

HOOF GROWTH

If a foot is shod, the length of wall will depend on the rate of hoof growth and the length of time between trimming and reshoeing. For the unshod horse, hoof length depends on

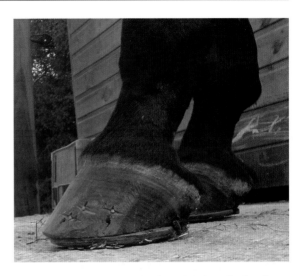

Fig. 64   Growth rings (the faint lines on the hoof) following the line of the coronary band and running parallel to each other.

whichever is the greater between the rate of growth or the rate of wear, and also to what extent the hoof wall splits and breaks away if it is allowed to become overgrown.

Both the rate of hoof growth and quality of hoof horn can be affected by local and systemic factors. Local changes such as blood flow and pressure can alter growth in an individual foot, whereas the effect of environmental, dietary and metabolic factors is likely to be seen in all four feet. Factors that only alter the rate of growth – for example temperature – do not alter hoof shape and are only likely to be noticed by changes in the amount of hoof to remove at the farrier's routine visit. Even when a growth ring becomes more obvious, as an indentation and ridge, growth will often remain even around the foot and remain parallel with the coronary band. This can occur in an individual foot from an injury or disease affecting the pastern, and in all four feet after a systemic infection or toxic condition. Single or multiple indentations are seen in feet, attributed to changes in grass growth ('grass rings'), being a common finding in horses and ponies out on grass, but are often likely to be due to metabolic changes in the horse; these will be discussed further with insulin resistance in Chapter 8 and 'IR rings' in Chapter 9.

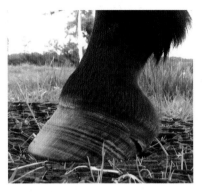

Fig. 65 Left fore of a New Forest pony kept out on grass (muzzled some of the time). The more obvious growth rings are commonly referred to as 'grass rings'.

There are some situations where there is a different rate of growth around a foot, when the rings no longer run parallel and there is divergence in the lines of growth. By far the most common situation where this occurs is in the feet of those horses suffering from chronic laminitis, when the spaces between the lines on the dorsal wall are narrower than at the heels. This is attributed to pressure from the extensor process of P3 on the coronary blood supply of the dorsal wall, following rotation of the bone, causing slower hoof growth. It occurs when the mechanical forces on P3 and the hoof have not been addressed correctly, and/or the underlying cause of laminitis has not been adequately controlled, for example with insulin resistance or PPID (*see* Chapters 7 and 8). In this situation, indentations in the wall may be referred to as 'laminitis rings', and are often accompanied by a change in angle of the dorsal wall.

When there is faster growth at the heel than at the toe, the longer the time between trims, the more upright the foot will become, which can only perpetuate the problem. Slower dorsal wall growth can also be a feature of the more severe club foot, where displacement of P3 occurs due to the mechanical forces from the DDFT.

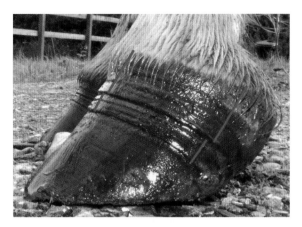

Fig. 66 Chronic laminitis. The ridge furthest down the wall is when laminitis occurred initially in this Welsh pony foot. As the problem continued a difference in the rate of growth occurred between the toe and the heel (Note similar ridges present on the right fore also.)

There are occasions when divergence of growth rings is due to faster-than-normal growth of part of the hoof. This is seen on new hoof growth following loss of part of the hoof wall from resection or injury, when the area not under pressure grows at a faster rate than the rest of the hoof wall and the rings are more widely spaced. However, because the faster growth is on the part of the wall that is unloaded, it will have no effect on the angle of the foot.

FOOT TRIMMING

With a uniform template (P3), and in most cases, even growth around the wall, a horse's hoof angle is greatly dependent on how the foot is trimmed. The way individual farriers and trimmers trim the feet will depend on how they were instructed, and how their own experience has changed this, taking into account the following:

- Their personal preference and opinion of what a normal shape and angle should be

- The type of horse and what it is used for
- How the horse moves
- Changes of wear that have occurred to the foot or shoe since the last trim
- Any conformational faults
- If there is any deformity or imbalance
- Whether a shoe is to be applied, or not
- Whether there is a specific trim for a certain type of shoe
- The environmental conditions
- Any request from the owner for a specific requirement or particular dislikes
- Any instruction from the vet

For the farrier, the same considerations have to be made for the choice of shoe that he applies.

Individual farriers trim feet to their image of a 'normal' foot and for their method of shoeing, with some farriers regularly leaving a higher heel and some trimming to a lower angle. Unfortunately this is not always to the benefit of the horse's feet and can sometimes be more to do with keeping the shoe on, which pleases the owner but may not be good practice. Provided there is a positive palmar angle (the angle between the solar border of P3 and the ground) and there is a straight HPA, many horses cope well with these different angles, but may require a different shoe type to do so.

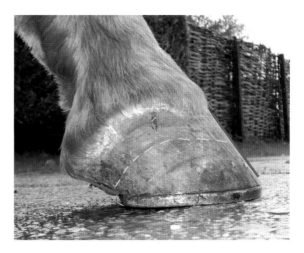

Fig. 67   It has taken the farrier some time to produce this misshapen foot, but the shoe stays on! The growth rings continue to grow parallel to the coronary band.

The Effect of Hoof Strength on the Hoof Angle

In order to change the hoof angle of a foot by trimming, the heels have to be trimmed either relatively more than the toe to produce a lower angle, or relatively less than the toe for a higher hoof angle. Because of the proximity of the tip of P3 to the ground, the amount of toe

---

BREAKOVER

The last phase of the stride is referred to as the 'breakover', and covers the time between the heel leaving the ground and the toe leaving the ground – between 'stance' when the foot is loaded, and 'lift' when the foot leaves the ground. 'Delayed breakover' means that this phase takes longer, as may be the case with a long toe, and 'shortened breakover' means that it takes less time. This might also be referred to as 'improved breakover' since it refers to a reduction in the forces acting on the dorsal wall and toe, and either means shortening of the toe, or providing a means for the foot to roll over more easily, and may thus be referred to as 'easing the breakover'.

There is some confusion as to what the 'point of breakover' refers to. It can be used to refer to the point on the toe that is the last part to leave the ground, but sometimes is used to refer to the point on the wall where the foot starts to roll over as the heel lifts off the ground. This point will be the same in a foot that does not have a roll on the toe from rounding the edge of the hoof or shoe (Figs 64 and 67).

that can be removed to provide a higher hoof angle is limited, so this is generally achieved by removing relatively less at the heels. This will have the required effect in stronger-walled hooves but is less likely to be successful in the weak-walled foot. Weaker feet are already struggling to maintain heel height and will often not be strong enough to support this extra heel length. They already have some heel collapse with horn tubules growing towards the horizontal, and leaving more heel may well cause them to collapse further.

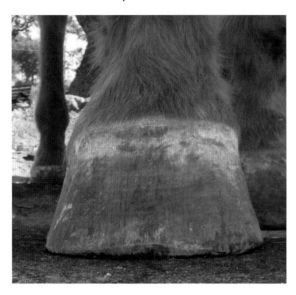

Fig. 68   Medio-lateral balance is assessed by examining the foot from in front (and from behind). Right fore foot.

If a lower hoof angle is achieved by trimming relatively less off the toe, breakover (*see* box) will be delayed, and the forces at the toe and on the dorsal wall will increase. Although a delay in breakover will also occur if the hoof angle is lowered by trimming more off the heels, the dorsal wall will be less liable to deform due to the shorter toe length. Some care needs to be taken not to remove too much heel at one time from a strong-walled upright foot so as to allow

the soft tissues, the deep digital flexor muscle and tendon in particular, to compensate for the change in forces on them – in the same way that a lady who wears high heels all the time may have discomfort when she changes to wearing low-heeled shoes.

Medio-Lateral Balance

The lateral (outer) side of the foot is often not an exact mirror image of the medial (inner) side, which tends to take more load and be slightly more upright. The line of the tubules at the toe should be straight down the wall and not angled over to one side, and the coronary band across the front of the foot should be level, with any curvature centred in the midline. Heel height should also be the same on both sides, and when the horse moves, it should land evenly on the foot.

Whereas dorso-palmar foot balance (hoof angle) commonly affects limb position rather than the reverse, it is often variations in conformation that affect medio-lateral balance of the foot, by altering the horse's action and thereby causing uneven foot-landing.

FOOT IMBALANCE

It is important not to get too carried away with analysing hoof form because horses have a great ability to cope with less-than-perfect feet, and even though they can have a hoof shape that is not apparently 'normal', can go through their career without these ever causing a problem. However, feet that aren't balanced are more likely to eventually cause lameness, so identifying any deformity and the reason it is there, will hopefully allow alterations to be made to avoid it becoming a problem.

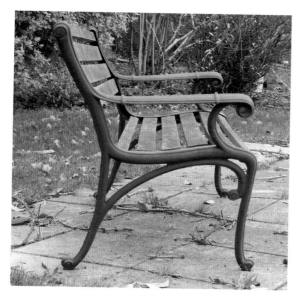

Fig. 69   Always look at the feet from all angles...

stretching is reduced and your muscles can relax again.

Although the coffin joint allows a reasonable amount of lateral movement, the pastern and fetlock joints do not, and pressure on the joints, due to imbalance, is likely to cause discomfort. The horse may be able to find a more comfortable stance by positioning the foot differently, or it may have to change the position of the leg to do so.

Hoof Deformation from Uneven Loading

Many factors can affect how feet land and load, but how a hoof distorts depends on the strength of the hoof wall, the direction of the uneven forces, and whether there is an intact laminar connection. The factors that cause abnormal loading include:

● Poor conformation
● The horse's action is not straight
● Unbalanced trim
● The type and position of the horse's shoe
● Uneven ground surface

Hoof distortion will be made worse by increased loading, in particular by the hoof size-to-weight

Static Balance or Imbalance

A horse that is not standing evenly on its legs may be doing so because it is in pain from an injury, but equally this might just be because of a foot imbalance. A horse will position its foot, if not always in the most comfortable position, at least in one that does not cause it discomfort: because of this, it will tend to position its leg in the direction of the highest part of an unbalanced foot.

A little experiment might help you understand what I mean: if you stand with the edge of a book under one side of your foot, your normal 'square' stance now becomes uncomfortable, but not one that would be considered painful. When you load the foot, you will be aware of the ankle joint stretching on the opposite side from the wedge, and what is normally a relaxed stance now becomes one where some of the muscles of the leg have become tense. If you now move the book and foot in the direction of the side that is raised, and then evenly load both feet, the joint

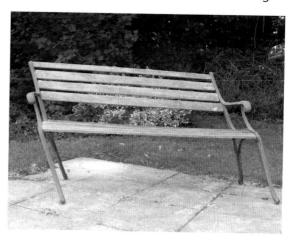

Fig. 70   ... Things may not be as they first appear.

ratio, the weight the horse carries when it is ridden, and the type and speed of the horse's work. The factors affecting how they distort include:

- Hoof strength
- Length of foot
- Wet or dry conditions
- How the foot is trimmed
- Laminitis

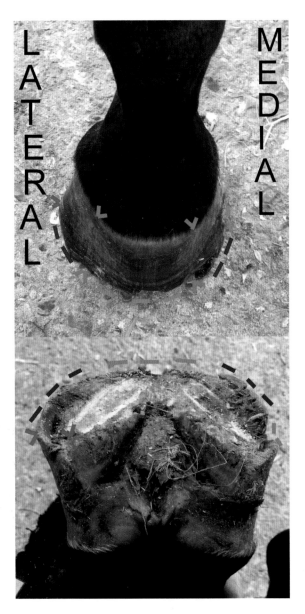

The hoof wall maintains its position relative to the other structures of the foot by its strong internal attachment to the dermal laminae, and its connection to the sole via the white line. The strength of the wall affects the way that uneven forces are spread to the rest of the hoof, and to the internal structures attached to it.

The hoof must withstand the initial forces of impact and then deal with the complex forces involved when the foot is loaded. If the foot lands unevenly, the part with the initial ground contact will be subjected to greater impact and vibration, but there will be greater load taken on the side of the foot that lands last, as the weight is thrown on to it. Loading of the hoof beyond its limits of compensation causes it to deform over time, but because the hoof is constantly growing, if the foot can be trimmed to even the load, this will often allow the new horn to grow down in a more normal way and a hoof deformity to grow out. However, continuous uneven forces on P3 can cause it to remodel, thus changing the underlying 'template' for hoof growth, and the likelihood of being able to correct these feet will inevitably be limited.

Distortion in the Sagittal Plane

The distribution of forces in the foot is complex, but the forces in the sagittal plane (front to

Figs 71a and 71b   Right fore of Thoroughbred yearling (fifteen months). The foot has become overgrown and the distal wall has flared (dotted blue line), and in doing so has started to cause distortion of the whole hoof capsule, with folding at the heel quarters and bending of the bar as the heel starts to turn under (red arrow heads), as well as folding in of the wall above the toe quarters (green arrow heads). The wall has broken away at the toe and at the fold of the medial heel quarter (orange dotted line). Regular trims can keep these changes under control.

back, parallel to the line of the body) are evidently the most significant, as seen by the frequency of deformation of the dorsal hoof wall (also the initial site of separation in cases of laminitis, *see* Chapter 7). The easiest way to work out the forces acting on the hoof is to study the weakest feet and observe how they deform. These deformities might include:

● Flaring of the hoof wall
● A marked difference between hoof angle and heel angle
● Collapsed heels, ranging from a slight turn-in of the heels to the situation where hoof growth is virtually horizontal
● A fold in the hoof wall at the heel quarter where the heel turns under
● Bars that are curved and lying close to the horizontal
● The sole flattening out and losing its concavity

This can be recognized as the end result, but it is hard to say whether it is the toe that flares first, the heels collapse first, or just that everything fails together.

One opinion would be that a horse landing on heels that are too weak causes them to collapse, and as the heels and bars fold, the dorsal wall angle lowers and increases the forces on the toe, as breakover is delayed. These breakover forces act not in the direction of the tubules but more across them, causing them to bend and the wall to flare. As the wall flares, the edge of P3 loses support from the white line/sole 'ledge', which leaves the bone sitting lower inside the hoof capsule (distal descent) and causes the sole to flatten (*see* Chapter 6).

If flaring extends around the foot to the heel quarters, the weak heels lose the support of the hoof acting as a unit as the heel quarters fold and the heels collapse further. However, it could be that the process starts with a weak dorsal

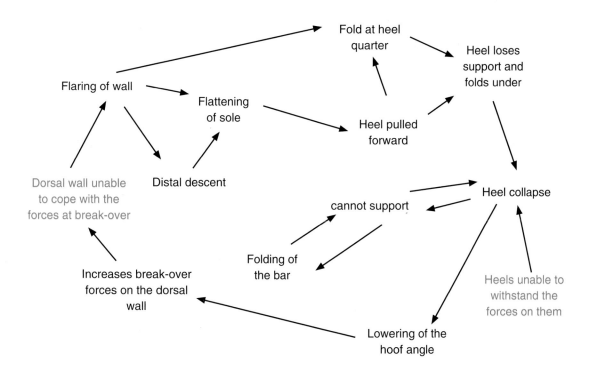

Fig. 72 *Factors contributing to the distortion of the weak-walled foot.*

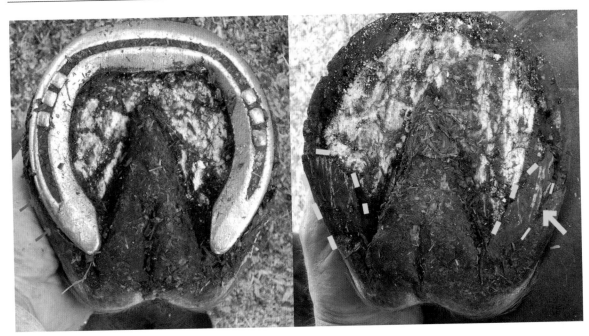

Fig. 73   A delay in re-shoeing, so the shoe is no longer supporting the wall (red arrows) and the overgrown heels have completely collapsed. The medial heel has folded under and is growing horizontal, and the lateral heel wall has bent and cracked (yellow arrow).

wall that flares, followed by flattening of the sole and folding at the heel quarter, whereupon the heels and the bars fold and collapse. Whatever starts the process, the way that weak feet deform always compounds the problem.

The Stronger Foot

An indication of hoof strength can be gained by looking at a foot from the side and assessing how it has distorted, and by observing any deviation of the dorsal wall and the extent of any heel collapse, as shown by the difference between the hoof and heel angles and the curvature of the coronary band. A foot with stronger horn can maintain its shape better, and this is most evident with the very strongest hooves that don't distort: they keep growing in the direction they are trimmed, so the heel will grow at the same angle as the dorsal

wall, and the coronary band down the sides of the foot will remain straight (*see* Fig. 62). However, although the strength and rigidity of these feet mean they are able to resist external forces, because of their limited ability to distort or expand they may not be so effective at compensating for internal force changes.

In slightly less strong hooves, the wall becomes flared only if the foot is overgrown, the heels will remain upright but at a lower angle than the dorsal wall, and there is some curvature to the coronary band. These features become more obvious in those feet with weaker walls, and although the extent of any changes is dependent on the uneven forces on the hoof capsule, the weaker the feet the more liable they are to distort, with deviation occurring higher up the wall as well as further round the foot.

When the heels turn under, the angle of growth of the horn tubules becomes lower, and this accounts for the curving of the coronary band; the curvature of the coronet increases as the difference between the heel and dorsal wall angle increases. In some cases, the coronary groove at the top of the wall becomes more vertical, which increases this curvature. In these feet, the size of the bars appears to contribute to this by increasing the internal pressures when the foot is weighted, causing the collateral cartilages to press against the coronary groove to make this more upright (*see* Chapter 6).

Some feet, at first glance, appear to flare from mid-way down the dorsal wall, but the proximal wall is actually bending inwards (*see* Chapter 12). This generally occurs when the toe is long in a relatively strong upright foot, where the strength of the heels and bars limits the foot's ability to expand to compensate for forces on the dorsal wall from the long toe.

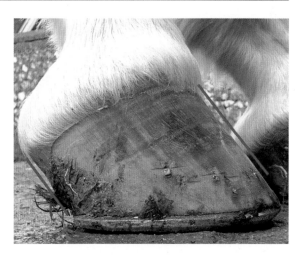

Fig. 74 Right fore of an Arab ×. A strong foot that is able to maintain similar heel and hoof angles.

High and Low Feet

Sometimes a horse's two front feet have obviously different hoof angles, in which case each foot needs to be assessed to identify which, if either, is normal. Not surprisingly, this is sometimes referred to as 'high/low foot syndrome'. The difference in shape may have started when the horse was a foal, and may be related to 'lateralized' behaviour, when one leg is consistently placed forwards when the foal is eating grass. At this stage the legs are relatively long compared to the rest of the body so the foal's head can't reach the ground without the limbs being placed wide apart. Those foals that consistently place the same leg forwards do seem to develop with this foot at a lower angle, whilst the leg positioned back develops as a more upright foot, and this difference quite often continues into adulthood.

Another suggestion for this foot combination is that the horse has a structural difference in limb length. This is a problem identifiable in

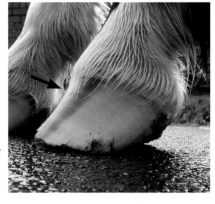

Fig. 75 Welsh Cob left fore. The angle between the coronary band and the top of the dorsal wall is less than normal because the hoof wall is bending inwards towards P3 below the extensor process (arrow).

people by measuring the distance from the hip to the ankle, but it is far more difficult to prove in the horse because, rather than having a straight leg to measure, a horse stands with its shoulder and elbow (and hip and stifle) in partial flexion, as well as its fetlock in dorsal flexion. It is probably more likely that, rather than a structural disparity in limb length, it is a functional one caused by an alteration of limb position due to a problem higher up the leg. Horses that are lame from a long-standing

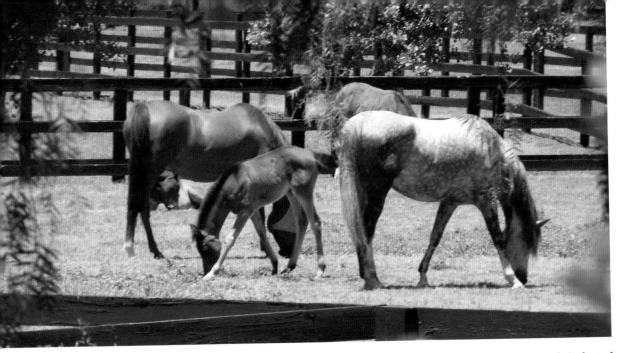

Fig. 76 'Lateralized behaviour' – consistent placement of the limbs when grazing as a foal may result in feet of a different shape.

problem – for example, arthritis in a joint – will often develop a more upright foot on that leg, due to reduced loading. When upper limb

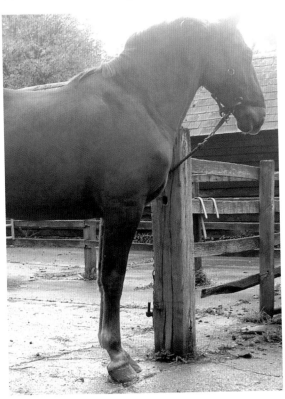

displacement is less obvious and the horse is not apparently lame, it is far more difficult to tell whether high/low feet are the result of an injury, or are the cause of the displacement, bearing in mind that limb position is often different with hooves of different angles (to maintain a straight HPA).

Whatever the cause for the disparity, the difference is often perpetuated by farriers, who continue to trim and shoe the feet differently. In some cases, the feet may become far closer in shape when hoof care is taken over by another farrier or trimmer, but any 'correction' is less likely if the foot changes are of long standing, because of bone remodelling.

Medio-Lateral Imbalance

Sometimes medio-lateral imbalance of the foot is easy to see, the more obvious signs being a sloping coronary band when looking at the foot

Fig. 77 A high- and low-angled foot with an even leg alignment might indicate limbs of a different length.

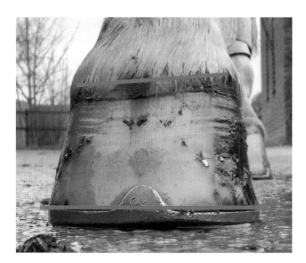

Fig. 78 *Medio-lateral imbalance in the left fore of this Welsh Cob, with the coronary band higher on the lateral side.*

also subjected to forces at an angle to the line of the tubules as the load shifts to the other side of the foot. Depending on the length and strength of the hoof, flaring may well occur on the side of impact, and because the hoof acts as a unit, as one side flares then the other side will tend to become more upright.

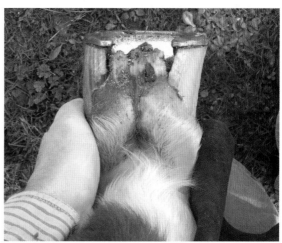

Fig. 80 *Welsh pony with an overgrown foot. It has a deviation of the lateral wall (on the right) and the medial wall has followed it.*

from in front, and angling of the dorsal wall tubules to one side rather than being vertical. Imbalance between the two sides of the foot may just be because the foot has not been trimmed level, but more commonly results from the way the foot lands due to the horse's conformation and action.

Any deviation from the perpendicular, or rotation of the limb, is likely to affect the horse's action and the way the feet land. The side of the foot that impacts the ground first is then

Medio-lateral imbalance can occur alone, or it may be in combination with dorso-palmar changes, in which case the situation becomes far more complicated. If a horse lands on the lateral toe-quarter, a greater load is passed over to the medial heel as the foot is weighted. Any flaring of the toe-quarter accentuates the uneven landing, and in a weak foot the medial heel collapses, and in a stronger foot the medial heel is shunted upwards. This displacement makes the two heels different heights, and is referred to as 'sheared heels'.

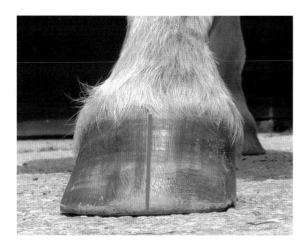

Fig. 79 *Yearling Welsh pony right fore. The horn tubules are deviating laterally.*

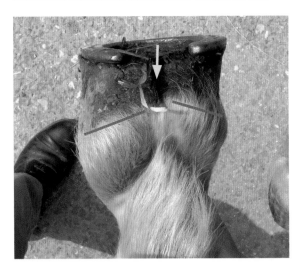

Fig. 81 Sheared heels in a Welsh Cob. Because of the different movement of the two heels, sheared heels are commonly accompanied by a deep central frog sulcus that can even extend back to cause a split in the skin between the heel bulbs.

ASSESSING AND CORRECTING FOOT DISTORTION

Any foot with a distortion should be assessed from all sides, including its solar surface, to try and work out exactly what is happening. A number of factors need to be considered when trying to correct a deformed foot.

As we have seen, having an understanding of how hooves of different strength deform will make it easier to identify changes early on, what forces are likely to have caused the deformation, and what might be the best way to correct it. It can also help us understand that there may be limitations as to what some feet are capable of dealing with, and that they may not be able to stand up to the level of work being asked of the horse. In some cases we may have to accept that control of a problem is all that is likely to be achieved.

As already discussed, the conformation of the horse will affect its action and can result in uneven forces acting on the hoof structure.

The balance of a horse's feet can also affect the way it moves and how the feet land, and whatever the horse's conformation, trimming the feet so that they land evenly will generally help prevent distortion developing and is likely to help reduce any distortion that has occurred. We have also noted that the greater the forces acting on the foot, the more likely it is that the hoof will become distorted, particularly when the forces are uneven. The forces on the feet increase when a horse is doing faster work, if it is carrying the extra weight of a rider, or even if the horse itself is overweight.

Since any hoof changes that have already occurred can alter how the foot breaks over and lands, they may exacerbate any deformity, so should be addressed as soon as they are noticed.

THE PROBLEMS INHERENT IN CORRECTION

Once the hoof wall has flared, the heels have collapsed and the tubules bent, correcting the problem can be extremely challenging. These changes may have been brought about by inappropriate hoof care and shoeing but, to get into this situation, the hoof will be weak and this lack of wall strength makes it that much more difficult to actually reverse.

The aim has to be to reduce the forces on the bent tubules of the flared wall and on heel tubules that have turned under. The amount of support provided by bent tubules will be limited, and if they continue to be loaded, they have no alternative but to bend even more. Trimming the hooves back to where the tubules are straighter and unloading the affected area are the aims of any correction, but there are practical problems in achieving this. Although trimming has less effect on hoof angle because of the horizontal nature of horn growth, with the sole already nearer the

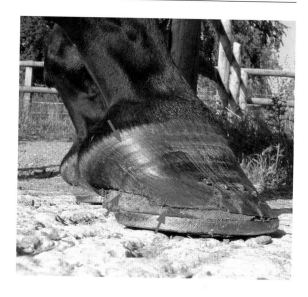

Fig. 82   The wedge under this shoe is obviously not helping this collapsed Thoroughbred foot. The heel has folded under behind the heel quarter (blue arrowhead), with the wall in front of this overlapping the pad (green arrow), so that the heel behind it is taking the weight and being compressed further (orange arrow).

ground, correction has to be done over a period of time to avoid making the horse footsore. This means that there always has to be a period of accommodation in the process before any correction is achieved, and vets, farriers and trimmers have a number of ways they use to try to deal with the problem.

An ordinary plain shoe fitted to the perimeter of the foot often causes the problem, particularly when left short at the heels, and can only make things worse. Some may try using a different type of shoe, sometimes with pads or wedges underneath them, whereas others will try to deal with the problem without shoes, maybe with the additional help of hoof boots or hoof casts (Equicast): each method has its advantages and disadvantages. If shoes are taken off feet like this, the horse will almost inevitably be foot-sore initially, which will limit how much hoof can be removed at a trim, and will be a problem if the owner wants to keep the horse in work. Dealing with the problem with more frequent, smaller trims and using hoof boots, or the casts, should help to keep the horse sound.

Shoes raise the soles off the ground, generally keeping the horse sound, but trimming is limited to when the horse is re-shod, and increasing the frequency puts more nail holes into the wall to weaken it further. Breakover is improved by having a rounded edge on the ground surface of the shoe, with some designed to be set back under the toe – such as the Natural Balance shoe – and if barefoot, by rounding the edge of the hoof wall. Applying artificial aids, such as wedges or a composite material, to the heels will raise the hoof angle but will ultimately fail if the tubules remain bent because they will continue to grow forwards and the heels will remain collapsed. Fibre-glass supports fixed to the heel walls have been used on some racing Thoroughbreds to strengthen the heels, and may help to prevent collapse, but are unlikely to be of any benefit once this has occurred. 'Quarter relief' describes the process when slightly more hoof is removed at the ground surface of the quarters, mimicking a finding in the feet of wild mustangs, but it is not suitable in this type of foot unless the bars can be trimmed in a way that provides adequate support, otherwise the heels are liable to collapse even more.

Environmental conditions can affect hoof strength and flexibility, and feet are more liable to distort if they are constantly wet. Constantly standing in wet and muddy ground therefore also makes correction more difficult, and providing the opportunity for the feet to dry out in order to regain rigidity is usually necessary if any collapse is to be reversed.

5 Upright Feet

I consider a foot with a hoof angle over 55 degrees to be an upright foot. 55 degrees is higher than the average hoof angle found in several studies of domesticated horses, but has been found to be the average hoof angle in some studies of feral horses. An angle over 55 degrees is only achievable if the hoof has sufficient strength for the heels to stay upright, because in weaker hooves the heels fold under and collapse.

It is generally easy to see what is meant when 'medio-lateral' imbalance is talked about, when there is a difference between the two sides of a foot, but it is not so easy to understand what vets mean when they talk about 'dorso-palmar'

balance or imbalance. It appears that these terms are used to refer to whether a horse has a straight hoof-pastern axis (or not). This opinion is often given when a foot has been placed for a radiograph, with the cannon in a vertical position and the HPA broken forward, but what appears to be 'normal' for these horses is for them to 'stand under', with the cannon angling backwards. In Chapter 3 I suggested that a horse is likely to change its stance to find a comfortable position if its foot is unbalanced, and it usually does this by altering its foot placement in the direction of the high part of the foot.

This also seems to be the response for horses

Figs. 83a and 83b A 'normal' stance for this cob gelding, with a hoof angle of about 57 degrees.

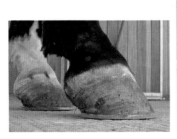

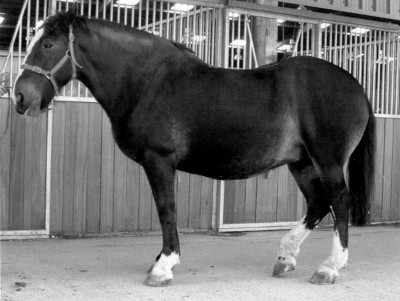

with upright feet, the high part being the heels in these cases. A study of the effect of raising the hoof angle on coffin joint pressure by applying wedges under the heels, showed that this caused a significant increase in pressure in this joint. This study used a cadaver leg placed with the cannon perpendicular, and it seems likely that if a horse with upright feet were to stand square it would find this increase in joint pressure uncomfortable. I believe this is why they 'stand under', rather than 'unloading painful heels', as some people suggest, although this might also be the case in some instances.

Something that is more likely to identify discomfort or pain in the heel area (palmar foot) is if a horse lands obviously toe first on a foot. By landing toe first, the horse is able to avoid fully weighting the heel if this action causes him discomfort. When landing toe first, the stride length will inevitably be shorter than when landing with the foot flat or the heel first (try this yourself). This action may be seen with the low-angled foot, where the collapsed heel might cause bruising or corns (*see* Chapter 9) – although it may also occur in horses suffering with navicular disease, with any shape of foot (*see* Chapter 11).

Specific foot conditions seem to be less commonly associated directly with upright feet than those with a low hoof angle and collapsed heels, but problems are likely to occur from limited movement of the hoof capsule, and from its reduced ability to compensate for forces of unequal loading. It would be hard to attribute a greater frequency of acute injury to the upright foot, but there would appear to be an association with some more chronic changes, for example ringbone, sidebone and even navicular disease.

THE CLUB FOOT

'Club foot' is a term used to describe a

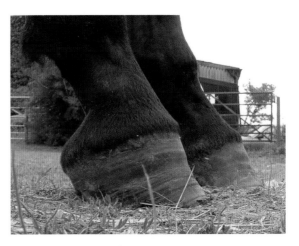

Fig. 84 A club foot, with a high hoof angle and broken-forward HPA. (This horse stood with a perpendicular cannon.)

foot which is abnormally upright, but it is also loosely used to refer to any foot with a noticeably greater hoof angle than the opposite foot. Although some attempts have been made to define a 'club foot' as well as to classify the severity, there appear to be anomalies in these definitions and classifications.

Features of a Club Foot

Bilateral club feet occur only rarely, so there is generally an obvious difference between the hoof angles of the two feet, with the club foot having a hoof angle over 60 degrees, and sometimes significantly more. Certainly if both front feet are upright they could both be club feet, but some farriers regularly shoe horses this way, so it would be as well to check other horses that they shoe.

A particular feature accompanying a club foot is the tightness of the deep digital flexor muscle and its associated tendon (DDFT). Attempts made to significantly reduce the hoof angle by trimming the heels will result in the heels not being able to touch the ground. This may not be known until it is tried, but the ability of a horse to alter its stance to maintain a straight HPA is a good indication that heel height can be reduced to some degree. Reducing the heel height of a very upright foot should always be done slowly, over a number of trimmings, to allow the muscle-tendon units and the internal structures of the foot to adapt to the new position.

A horse with a club foot generally stands square (with a vertical cannon) and a broken forward HPA. Note that radiographs taken of any upright foot, with the horse's leg positioned with the cannon vertical, will show a broken-forward HPA, and they do not differentiate between horses able to alter their stance ('upright foot'), and those that cannot ('club foot').

Similarities with Laminitis

Some other features of a club foot have similarities with changes seen in the feet in chronic laminitis. A very common feature of chronic laminitis is a different rate of hoof growth around the wall, with faster growth at the heels than at the toe, identified by divergence of the growth rings around the hoof, and this is also seen in some club feet. Demineralization and remodelling of the tip of P3 is evident on radiographs of more severe club feet, and this also occurs commonly in chronic laminitis.

Deviation of the dorsal wall occurs in both conditions; with the club foot generally having curvature ('dishing'), whereas a change in the line of the wall in laminitis is generally associated with an obvious growth ring and, significantly, the angle between the top of the hoof wall and the coronary band, is more likely to be 95 degrees in the club foot than the 105 degrees normally found in chronic laminitis (*see* Chapter 12), which helps to differentiate between the two conditions.

Note that some medium to strong feet

with high heels and the toe left long can have dishing of the dorsal wall (*see* Chapter 4), but these can be returned to a better shape if the heels are trimmed and the toe brought back in order to ease the breakover.

Problems Associated with a Club Foot

Club feet often have stress damage to the dorsal laminae, and increased pressure on the sole from the tip of P3. They are less able to compensate for the forces acting on them due to the constant tension in the DDFT, and even if the club foot is classed as less severe, it will undoubtedly limit a horse's athletic potential. With the obvious difference in hoof angle between the front feet, inevitably there must be a difference in the way the feet are loaded, and the horse is likely to move differently on the two legs, and thus potentially have a greater chance of injury, regardless of the stress damage in the foot.

What Causes Club Feet?

Many club feet develop due to changes early in a foal's life, either with a congenital problem or as an acquired flexural deformity (*see* later in this chapter). Some of these can be corrected, or at least improved in the young horse, but if not dealt with at this stage, the opportunity to do so will have been lost due to bone remodelling and other changes that occur in these feet.

In the adult horse a foot can become very upright due to abnormal loading as a result of a problem higher up the leg, and it can also occur due to DDF muscle contracture as a consequence of foot pain in chronic laminitis. In laminitis, the foot may not appear upright if the unattached wall is allowed to grow forward, but the new growth at the top of the wall will be very upright. Although

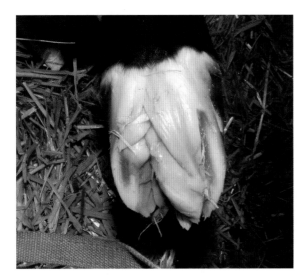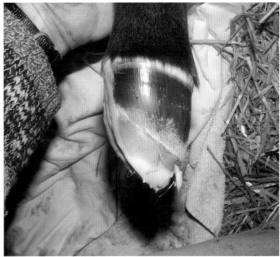

Figs. 85a and 85b   When a foal is born, each hoof has a retained cap of soft unpigmented horn covering its tip and bottom surface, which helped to protect the uterus from damage by the foetus. After birth these quickly dry, separate, and are shed as the foal walks around.

these present similar practical problems of management as other club feet, with the heels not reaching the ground if trimmed, the problems they present are rather different from club feet, which have a greater structural integrity.

The upright feet described so far refer to the front feet of adult horses, but there are feet that naturally have a higher hoof angle. First, foals' feet are more upright than those of an adult; then it is suggested that the feet of donkeys are 5 to 10 degrees higher than the front feet of adult horses; and finally in hind feet, P3 has a bone angle 10 degrees greater than those of the front feet.

FOAL FEET

Although functional straightaway, the immature foot of the newborn foal, which has developed in the weight-free environment of the uterus, has to adapt rapidly to cope with the increasing demands of foalhood. The foot structures have

to increase in size in line with the rapid growth of the foal, and must adapt to deal with its increasing weight and activity. At birth, the outer wall (stratum medium) is fully keratinized, but this is not the case for the rudimentary

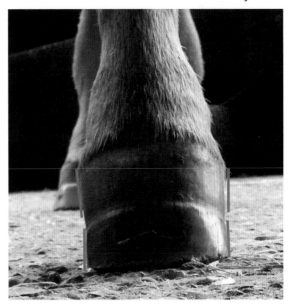

Fig. 86   Thoroughbred foal foot growing down; two months after birth.

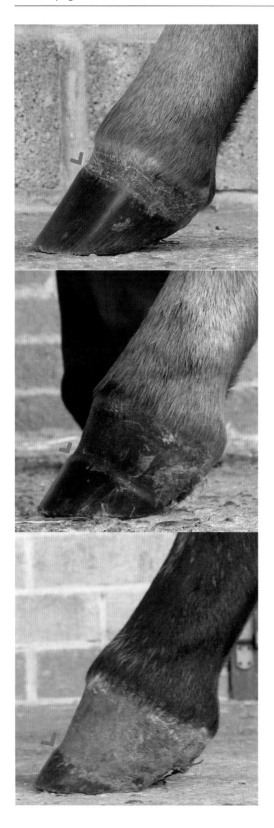

laminae of the stratum lamellatum. The basal cells of the primary lamellae proliferate, and combined with the development of secondary lamellae, the laminae increase in size and length, which is necessary for the foot to grow in size.

With increased stimulation, new horn grows down rapidly from the coronary band (15mm per month, as opposed to at most 10mm in adults) and the 'foal foot' grows out in around four months. The hoof angle of the 'foal foot' is initially about 55 degrees, but this angle becomes higher as new horn is produced from a coronary band that is increasing in size, up to 65 degrees or more. At birth the foot is pointed, being narrower at the ground surface than at the coronary band, and it continues to be this shape for several months after the foal foot has grown out, and will only start to have divergent side walls at nine to twelve months.

This is all occurring over a bone that is also increasing in size. In the foetus, P3 develops by bone being laid down (ossification) on a cartilage template, but it is not fully developed at birth. The bone increases in size by continuing to ossify cartilage, to form the palmar processes, and from new bone formed under the periosteum until P3 is fully formed. Abnormal forces on the developing bone can affect its shape for life.

Associated Limb Changes

Having evolved as 'potential prey', foals need to have a skeleton and supporting structures sufficiently developed to allow them to be up and running with their dam almost immediately. It is not uncommon, at birth,

Fig. 87 Thoroughbred left fore, the 'foal foot' growing out: a) one month, b) two months, c) three months after birth.

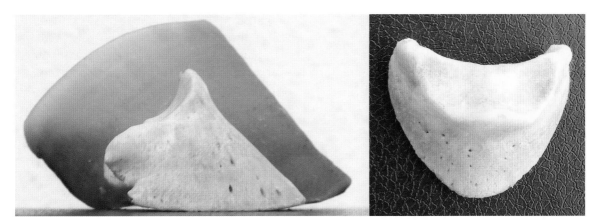

Fig. 88   Hoof and coffin bone of a foal. P3 has a curved solar border when seen from the side, and limited palmar processes.

for there to be some laxity (or tautness) of the supporting tendons and ligaments, and the newborn foal will often have limbs that are not straight – sometimes they are too upright, due to tightness of the tendons, or the fetlock is low due to flexor tendon laxity. The problem for an owner is to know when to be concerned, and when assistance is needed. However, provided the foal is able to get up and down relatively easily and can stand to suck, little needs to be done immediately since very many of these congenital limb problems will straighten up, without assistance, within a few days.

Nevertheless, if you are concerned that the foal has a possible limb deformity, the first thing to do is to compare the limbs. Then try to establish when the deformity developed – was it noticeable at birth, or did it develop later? Is it getting worse or improving? Does it affect the foal's stance and/or movement? *If in doubt, seek advice.* A photographic or video record of a foal's development can be extremely useful.

Uneven forces on growing long bones can cause them to distort, and these distortions will sometimes carry on to adulthood – for example, valgus of the carpus (knock knees)

and varus of the carpus (bow legs). Angular and flexural limb deformities alter the way the feet are loaded, and it may be possible to 'correct' limb abnormalities by foot trimming or by the application of an orthosis to the foot. (An orthosis is something applied to a foot or limb to help straighten it – orthotics is sometimes used, but this actually refers to the medical science of the manufacture and application of orthoses.) Early identification of limb deformities and, importantly, getting the foal used to being restrained and having its feet picked up (and trimmed) when young, will make it much easier for early intervention to be given to those that need it.

'Acquired' limb deformities can develop from different rates of growth in an epiphysis (growth plate) of a long bone. Damage to one side of the plate can result in slower growth, causing deviation of the distal end of the bone. Growth at the epiphysis is stimulated by compression, but is slowed if this compression is excessive or following injury. It has been suggested that this response allows some minor distortions to correct themselves, because if one side of the growth plate grows more slowly, it responds to the resultant increased compression on it by growing faster, and thus helps to straighten the deviation. Those with greater deviation may require surgery on the leg and/or the application of an orthosis to the foot for correction.

Ballerina Syndrome

Ballerina syndrome refers to a situation where an apparently normal foal changes, within a few days, to having very upright pasterns and walking on the tips of its toes. Some suggest that the speed of the bone growth is too fast for the tendons to adapt, but this explanation does not fit with the rapidity of the change. It seems more likely that it is initially a response to foot pain, and the flexor muscles contract in response to this, in an attempt to give some stability to the limb. With continuing pain, the muscle goes into contracture (continuous contraction), which itself is likely to be painful, and this accentuates the problem. With the muscles constantly contracted, the tightness in the DDFT is sufficient to hold the heel off

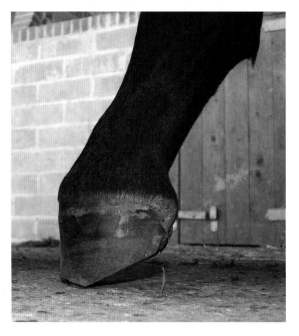

the ground, and the foal walks on its tip-toes like a ballerina.

Certainly in some cases the problem starts as the 'foal hoof' grows out, when there is just a small part of it left covering the toe. This pointed cap of horn becomes distorted and bends, and in doing so the tip of P3 loses its support and presses directly on the sole, causing pain (*see* Figs 87 and 89). A similar reaction to toe pain occurs in some cases of chronic laminitis, and in both situations what seems odd is that the response, by standing on the toe and not weighting the heel, seems very likely to just add to the pain.

Management of Ballerina Syndrome

In the first instance the aim must be to control the pain, to break the pain/contracture cycle, because only then can the muscle relax and lengthen to reduce the tension on the tendon. If the pain is due to loss of support at the toe, this area must be protected and supported.

There is obviously no point in trying to trim the heels since they already do not reach the ground. Initially the application of a wedge to the heel can help support the whole foot and reduce the discomfort; then as the muscle is able to relax and lengthen, the wedge can be reduced and then removed as things settle down. Mild cases may settle down just with restriction, pain relief and judicious trimming, but others may require a toe extension fitted to the foot to help stretch the muscle. Any

Fig. 89 Ballerina syndrome gets its name because the foal walks on the tips of its toes – the heel is not able to reach the ground (the flared toe has been rasped off in preparation for an orthosis). A Thoroughbred foal.

toe extension must be attached to the whole hoof to provide overall support, and will also provide protection to a painful toe. Stress damage to the foot and restriction of hoof growth are concerns when toe extensions are applied.

Some vets advise having a check ligament desmotomy (cutting the supporting ligament of the DDFT), or even a tenotomy (when the DDFT itself is cut). There could be situations when either of these is necessary, but very many cases will settle down without the need of this.

Generally the mare and foal will be stabled and the mare's food restricted, to try to slow the foal's speed of growth. Limiting the movement of the foal will help to reduce its pain, and if there is an orthosis attached to the foot, will help to protect the foot, as well as the foal itself, from being damaged by it.

It would seem sensible for thoroughbred foals that have suffered (and recovered) from ballerina syndrome not to be put into race training early. They are likely to need time for the muscle/tendon unit to lengthen sufficiently to be able to stand up to training, otherwise they will be more liable to 'break down' (strain their tendons).

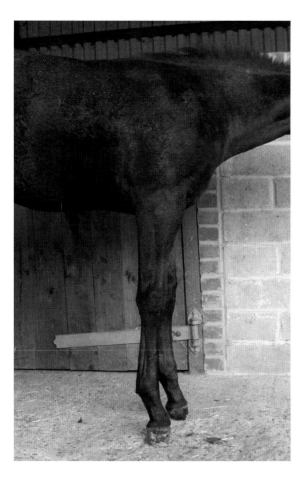 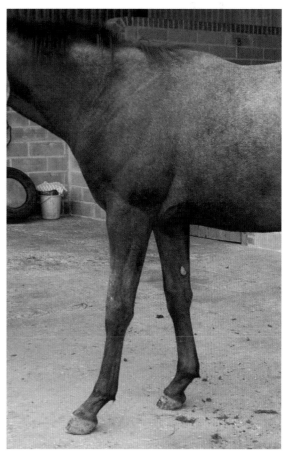

Figs. 90a and 90b   The same Thoroughbred as the preceding picture. These two photographs were taken exactly one year apart. The orthoses fitted in the left picture were not satisfactory and were replaced with toe extensions.

DONKEY FEET

Although the donkey's basic anatomy is the same, the shape and form of its hoof differs from that of the horse and pony. Their hooves are U-shaped, rather than being the rounder shape of horses, and the wall is relatively thicker than that of a pony of similar size, its thickness being consistent around the foot, rather than being thinner at the heels.

The tubule distribution through the thickness of the wall is also different, with donkey hooves having a broader inner stratum medium, with larger tubules and a less concentrated distribution. There is a greater moisture content in the hoof, and there are also fewer laminae than in the feet of horses, the overall result being that donkeys' hooves are more flexible than horses' hooves.

Although it is suggested, in the UK, that donkeys have a thicker sole than horses and that it should be in contact with the ground in the front third of the foot, working donkeys in the Middle and Far East, in an environment far more suited to them, generally have solar concavity and little, if any, sole contacting the ground (similar to horses).

In the normal donkey foot the dorsal wall is often more upright than in horses and ponies, and the upright side walls and heels give the feet their 'U'-shape. The hoof angle is reported to be 5–10 degrees higher than in horses and ponies, which is not actually very helpful since there is no agreement about what a horse's 'normal' hoof angle is. The principle that the best function of the distal limb occurs when the hoof-pastern axis is straight still applies to the donkey, and this should be the aim when trimming their feet.

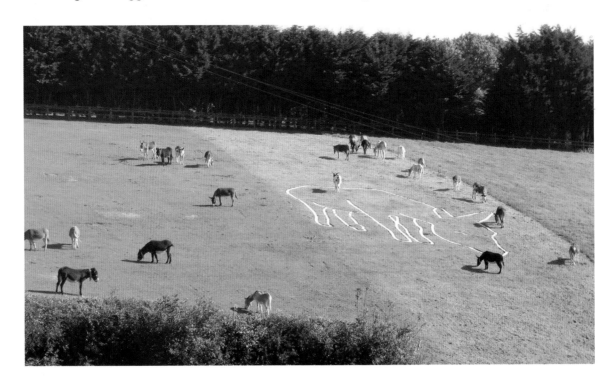

Fig. 91   The Donkey Sanctuary in Sidmouth, Devon, has a population of over 2,000 rescued donkeys, and the Sanctuary's experience and research makes them an excellent source of information on donkeys, including their feet.

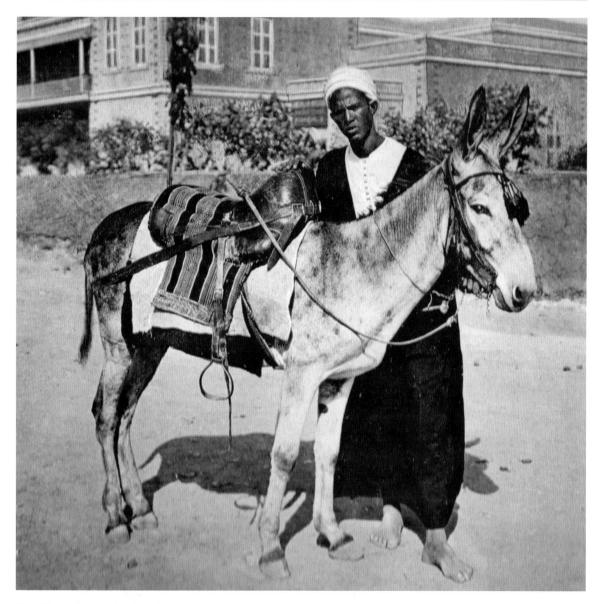

Fig. 92   A donkey (ass) with its owner in Egypt in 1910 (both barefoot).

It is difficult to describe what a 'normal' foot is for donkeys in the UK because the majority of them have abnormal feet, affected by laminitis or related problems. The reason for this is that the environment and conditions that we keep them in are so far removed from their natural situation. Donkeys (or more specifically asses) evolved in the arid conditions of North Africa, and had to travel over hard and stony ground in order to find food and water. This does not fit well with the quantity and type of food that is available here in the UK. As well as this, very few donkeys here are ever required to work, and this results in a population of insulin-resistant animals with the consequential hoof changes typical of laminitis and seedy toe. This will be discussed further in Chapter 8.

HIND FEET

The hoof and sole take the shape of the bone they cover, so that P3 in the hind feet produces a foot that is more pointed in shape, and has greater solar concavity than the front feet. However, the greater bone angle of P3 (55 degrees as opposed to 45 degrees) is not reflected in a significantly higher hoof angle because of the way that the front and hind feet are trimmed.

Forefeet are trimmed to give a positive palmar angle (*see* box), with a hoof angle generally somewhere between 47 and 57 degrees, whereas hind feet are far more

THE PALMAR/PLANTAR ANGLE

The angle between the solar border of P3 and the ground is called the *palmar angle* in the front feet, and the *plantar angle* in the hind feet.

When the palmar processes of P3 are higher than the tip of the bone (tipped forwards) the angle is referred to as a *positive* palmar/plantar angle.

When the tip of the bone is higher than the palmar processes (tipped back) the angle is referred to as a *negative* palmar/plantar angle.

When the solar border is parallel with the ground (P3 is ground-parallel) it is described as having a *zero* palmar/plantar angle.

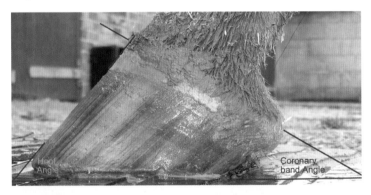

Fig. 93   Thoroughbred left hind foot.

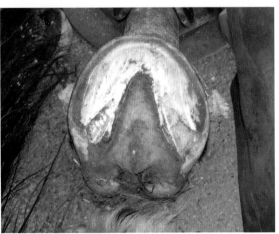

Fig. 94   Sole view of a Warmblood × left hind foot.

consistently trimmed with a 55-degree hoof angle and a close to zero plantar angle (ground-parallel solar border).

Although all four feet are involved in bearing weight and absorbing concussion, as well as in acceleration and deceleration, landing on the front feet requires them to be able to cope with greater concussion, and having a positive palmar angle helps them to deal with this. The hind feet, however, have a far greater role in propulsion and acceleration, with the power of the muscles of the hindquarters propelling the horse forwards by pushing off from the hind feet, and a zero plantar angle seems to be more suitable for this. The difference in hoof shape also reflects this: it is easier to land on an even round shape (as is more typical of the front feet), while the more pointed hind foot is better able to dig into the ground to maximize thrust, in the same way that human sprinters use starting blocks.

The Associated Stance

A 'normal' conformation for the hind leg is suggested as one where a vertical line dropping

However, whether tied up or loose, horses will far less frequently be seen standing square on their hind legs (with both legs aligned), so it is more difficult to judge a horse's hind limb conformation. Horses that are shown will commonly be trained to adopt a stance that lines up the limbs, sometimes with the hind limbs extended behind them, or even the exaggerated 'parked out' stance where the fore limbs are camped in front and the hinds are markedly camped behind. The suggestion is that this shows off the conformation of the horse, though in reality it only allows comparison of one limb against another, rather than an overall picture.

When wearing high heels (from observation only) ladies do not stand leaning forwards, but change their posture and remain upright, and this is the same for horses with higher

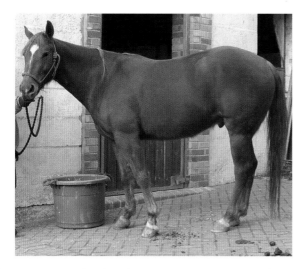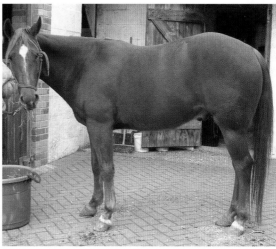

Figs. 95a and 95b   These two photos show the change in stance following trimming of the left hind foot, 'standing under' before the trim (left) and 'standing square' on that foot following it (right).

down from the tuber ischia of the pelvis (the most posterior bony prominence on each side of, and below the level of the tail) follows the line of the cannon bone, and is accompanied by a straight HPA (*see* Fig. 46).

hoof angles in their hind feet, rather than the unnatural show stance. Whereas a horse stands under on a front foot with a higher hoof angle, they do so on a hind foot with a low hoof angle (*see* Fig. 95).

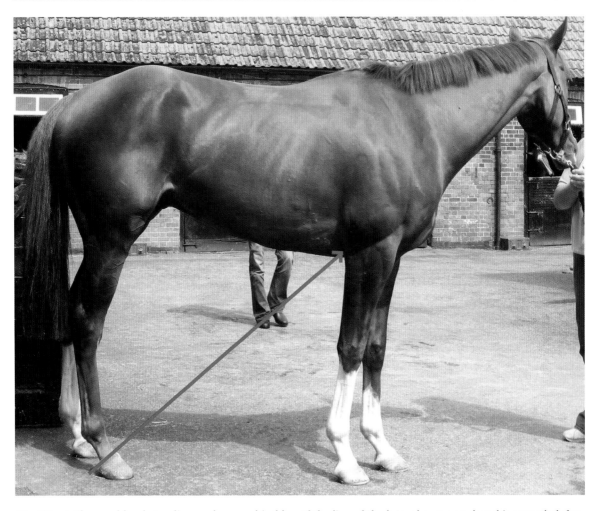

Fig. 96   A Thoroughbred standing under on a hind leg. If the line of the lateral coronary band is extended, for a foot with P3 at a negative plantar angle, this line will be close to the elbow, rather than closer to the back of the knee, which is the case when P3 is ground-parallel.

A negative plantar angle in hind feet can be estimated by visualizing where an extension of the line of the coronet would hit the front leg. Normally this line would end up at the middle of the forearm, but if P3 has a negative plantar angle it will reach the elbow (Fig. 96). Although actual measurement of this is not easy, a steeper angle of the coronary band to the ground (greater than 30 degrees), combined with the foot placed forwards under the body, is a very good indication of a negative plantar angle

of P3. Standing under on a hind foot doesn't always indicate this, and can occur if the foot is simply overgrown with a long toe, although in this case the coronet line will be at a normal angle (at 30 degrees).

Standing under may also be seen in the 'classic' laminitis stance, when both hind legs are placed under the body in an attempt to take weight off the front feet.

When soldiers stand to attention, their feet are turned out rather than straight, and although a horse's 'normal' hind limb position, from behind, is suggested as one where the leg follows a perpendicular line down from the tuber ischia, they too generally stand with their toes pointing out and the hocks slightly turned in. Where the hocks are turned in to an exaggerated degree, the horse is referred to as 'cow-hocked'.

Hind Limb Action

Forelimbs have a relatively straightforward action, with the legs moving forwards and back for flat foot placement in front of the horse; at faster speeds, when the forelimbs are not taking weight, they are tucked up under the chest before striding out again. For the hind limb it is rather more complicated, restricted as it is by being attached to the pelvis at the hip. The hind limb action is limited by the shape of the hip joint, and foot placement differs at different paces because of movement of the pelvis caused by rotation, flexion and extension of the

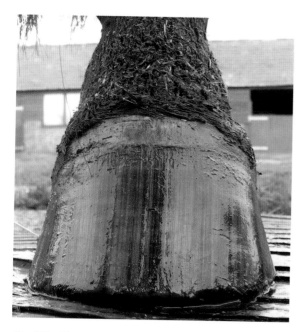

Fig. 97   Thoroughbred left hind foot.

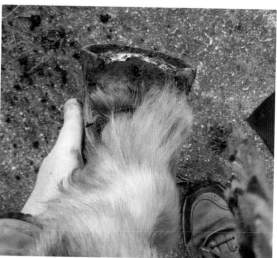

Fig. 99   ABOVE: Left hind foot of a New Forest pony × with the medial side higher on the image and the frog pointing axially.

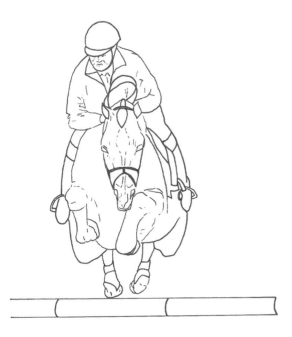

Fig. 98   LEFT: A showjumper: the forelimbs are folded up under the chest, but the hind limbs need to be abducted (away from the body) in order to get them up and out of the way.

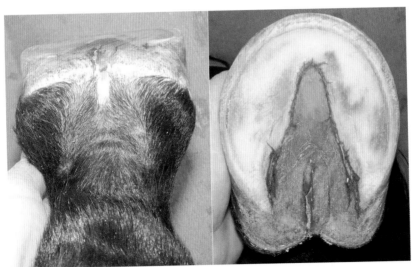

Fig. 100   Right hind foot of a Quarter Horse, showing an even foot, but at a slight angle to the pastern.

spine. As the hind limb is flexed, it also rotates so that the stifle moves outwards, avoiding the abdomen, and the lower part of the leg moves axially (towards the mid-line), and stays this way as the foot is extended forwards to land on the ground, giving better support for the horse than if it were to land on legs placed wide.

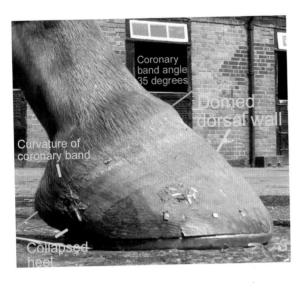

Fig. 101   Right hind foot of the Thoroughbred pictured in Fig. 96, showing a domed dorsal wall, collapse of the heel and curvature of the coronary band towards the heel. The angle of the coronary band (greater than 30 degrees) indicates that P3 is at a negative plantar angle in this foot.

When the hind limb is picked up and held behind the horse, the heels and bearing surface of the foot are not at right angles to the line of the cannon, as is generally the case for the forefoot, but at an angle that gives the impression of being higher on the medial side. The centre line of the frog aims slightly axially (inwards) from the line of the limb, but the two sides of the bottom of the foot are still generally even in shape.

This cannot just be attributed to different heel heights, since when trimmed right down to the level of the sole, the heels and frog are still not at right angles to the flexed pastern. When the foot is held up it appears to be in axial rotation (turned-in), but when the foot is on the ground it is abaxial, with the toe slightly turned out and the hock turned in to some degree. When moving, a foot of this shape allows the axially placed hind foot to land flat on the ground.

Hind Foot Deformation

As with front feet, the shape of hind feet and how they deform is dictated by the strength of the hoof horn: thus strong feet retain a straight dorsal wall, have heels of similar angle, and have limited deformity as they grow longer.

Weak hind feet rarely have flaring of the dorsal wall, and when overgrown, the wall typically becomes domed, commonly referred to as 'bull-nosed'. This occurs with some degree of heel collapse, the extent of which is related to hoof strength, but also to the type and severity of work and the method of shoeing.

The domed shape of the hind foot is often accentuated by wear of the toe, and by the way the foot is rasped in preparation for, or after, shoeing. There is obvious curvature of the coronary band accompanying the domed dorsal wall, and these feet have a tendency towards a negative plantar angle for P3 and greater solar concavity. As with front foot distortion, the change in dorsal wall direction occurs below the top 2cm (1in), the area of hoof growth.

The difference in the way that the dorsal wall of front feet and hind feet distort indicates that the hooves are subjected to different forces. Because the dorsal wall of a front foot deforms by flaring, the greatest forces of distortion must be when the foot is breaking over, whereas the dorsal wall of hind feet becomes domed (convex), indicating that it is the forces of landing and deceleration that are greatest. The reason is that this is the stance phase that is occurring on the front and hind feet when the weight of the horse is over the top of them. The front foot lands in front of the horse but breaks over underneath it, and the hind foot lands under the horse and breaks over behind it.

The firmness of the surface that a horse is working on will have an effect on whether different foot shapes or shoe types can position the hind legs to achieve maximum propulsion. On soft ground a pointed foot will sink into the ground to provide a larger surface area to push against, but on hard ground it will find it more difficult to get into a suitable position to push off. On firm ground a squarer toe or a set-back shoe will be better, though a long toe on this surface will quickly become squared off from wear.

A 'lazy' horse may square off the toes by

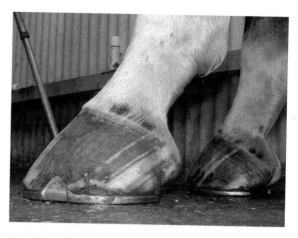

Fig. 102   *The hind feet of a Hanoverian showing domed dorsal walls ('bull-nosed'), marked curvature of the coronets, and a degree of collapse of the heels with a change in alignment of the wall tubules, as demonstrated by the line of the stripes on the walls.*

dragging its feet, but this can also occur with a physical or neurological problem. A squared-off toe on a single hind foot is likely to be due to a problem somewhere higher than the foot, when the horse struggles to bend the leg or move it forwards, but since all the joints are flexed together, identifying which part of the limb is affected may not be easy.

With a long toe, particularly if P3 has a negative plantar angle, the time between the heel lifting and the toe leaving the ground (the breakover) will be delayed, and with the foot not positioned so well for the horse to push off, is likely to increase the forces on other parts of the limb. Although there is no proven link between horses with a negative plantar angle and strains of the suspensory ligament (desmitis) or of the sacro-iliac ligament (that joins the pelvis to the spine), there does seem to be some circumstantial evidence to suggest this. Correcting the plantar angle and making sure breakover is shorter should help to prevent these problems.

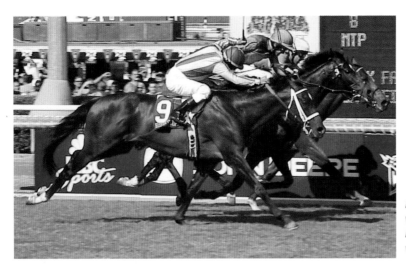

Figs. 103a and 103b   The horse's weight is over the hind foot when it lands, and over the front foot when it breaks over.

Medio-Lateral Imbalance

Because the hind foot is at a slight angle to the limb, it is more difficult to judge its medio-lateral balance, and the foot needs to be examined both on and off the ground, and the horse's stance and movement studied in order to assess this properly.

Although the dorsal wall becomes domed rather than flared, the way the rest of the hoof distorts is similar to a front foot. Weaker heels and bars fold under and collapse and may cause the heel quarters to fold. If this accompanies a domed dorsal wall, the wall may fold inwards at the toe quarters in between these bulging areas. A wall crack may develop here, but this would generally remain superficial, and only rarely extends to the deeper layers.

Due to the foot shape and the way that it lands, the most common deformity of a hind foot is one where the medial wall stays fairly upright and the lateral wall angle is lowered. There may be a flare to the lateral wall, but sometimes the change is due to an inward bend midway down the wall. The coronary band across the front of the foot is generally curved, but in these cases slopes down to the lateral side from the highest point above the medial toe quarter. If the difference is more marked,

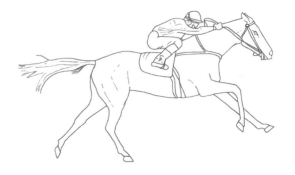

the foot may twist when walking, with the hock moving out (abaxially) after landing, as the limb straightens.

Occasionally the fold and flare is in the medial wall, and this is likely to be accompanied by the horse standing straight or toe in; when the foot is picked up, the frog points slightly out (abaxially), rather than in (axially), as is usually found.

Trimming and Shoeing

A horse may have shoes all round, but not infrequently only the front feet are shod and the hind feet are left bare. This is the policy of some riding establishments which turn out groups of horses together, to try to reduce the injuries

Fig. 104 The right hind of a hunter. There is flaring of the medial wall and a slight convexity of the lateral wall. This is the opposite from what is usually found, where the lateral wall is the one that flares.

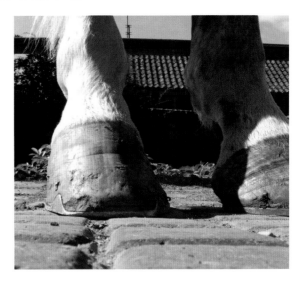

caused by kicks. Hind feet are generally shod with two quarter clips where horses are exposed to muddy conditions, to help retention of shoes – sometimes the shoe follows the shape of the toe, but often it is set back behind the point of the toe. This variation tends to be the way individual farriers shoe, rather than for what a particular horse is doing and the ground it is working on.

Probably the most significant deformity in the hind feet is the collapse of the heels, and the aim has to be to correct this, or at least to limit it. The reduced height of the heels when they have folded under can cause P3 to have a negative plantar angle, but even if the plantar angle is zero (ground-parallel), collapse of the heels contributes to the increased curvature of the coronary band and doming of the dorsal wall. Many of the folds in the wall will disappear if the heels can be made more upright and the foot lands evenly. If even foot-landing is achieved at the walk, provided the horse is sound, it will generally land level at faster paces, too.

6 The Palmar Structures

The palmar structures include the bars, the frog and the sole, and this chapter will discuss the role of these structures, and the possible problems associated with them.

THE BARS

The bars of the foot do not get the attention they deserve, and are often given only a few lines in books and articles. When looking at the bottom of the foot, it is difficult to visualize the extent of the bars or to work out their relationship to other foot structures, and therefore get an idea of their importance. Also, cadaver specimens are generally cut in ways that transect the bars, and this doesn't make interpretation of their position or role any easier.

It is simplest to think of the bars as the part of the hoof that, rather than completing the circle, has turned inwards at the angles of the heel. By doing this, the bars are still able to play their part in taking weight and providing a bearing surface, but they also allow movement of the back part of the foot while giving support to the heels and internal structures. The bars can be seen on the underside of the foot extending forwards from the angles of the heel alongside the frog. They follow their internal laminae down to the bearing surface as new horn is produced, and because the bar blends with the sole on its anterior (front) border, it is difficult to identify where the bar ends and the sole starts; however, there are internal and external features that help us to do so.

The bar has a similar construction to the hoof wall, and has the same strip of un-pigmented horn that can be seen when it is trimmed down. Internally, the extent of the bar is identified by where its laminae end, and the position of the navicular bone in relation to this is of particular significance.

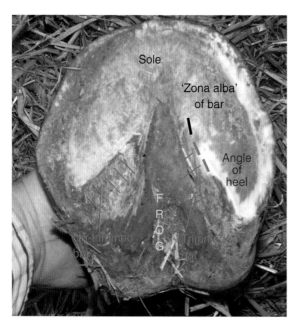

Fig. 105 Un-trimmed and trimmed bar on a Thoroughbred foot (right fore). The un-pigmented 'zona alba' can be seen on the trimmed bar (medial). In some texts 'zona alba' is used to refer to the 'white line', but in others (which includes this book) it refers to the unpigmented hoof wall – the inner stratum medium and the stratum lamellatum.

The Role of the Bars

It is easier to consider what happens when a foot is peripherally loaded on a hard, flat surface rather than on a softer one where loading is spread over the whole bearing surface of the foot. When weight is put on to a leg, dorsal flexion of the fetlock joint causes the pastern bones to descend towards the ground behind P3. The descent of the fetlock is limited primarily by the suspensory apparatus (the SDFT, DDFT and suspensory ligament) but also by a variety of ligaments, and for P2 and the navicular bone by structures inside the hoof. P2 descent is restricted by its lower (distal) end pushing against the collateral cartilages as it moves down between them, and depression of the navicular bone is limited by the structures in the foot that lie directly beneath it.

Any support given by the digital cushion will depend on how much fibrocartilage has been laid down in it, and only if, or when, the frog is in contact with the ground can its compression limit the descent of the navicular bone. It has to be the more rigid structures of the sole and anterior edge of the two bars beneath the navicular bone that consistently limits its downward movement.

The bar has its most rigid attachment on its posterior (rear) border, where it connects to the hoof at the angle of the heel. The bar corium on its proximal (top) border is straight and is attached to the corium of the frog, and its laminar corium, the sensitive laminae of the bar, is mostly attached to the base of the collateral cartilage. Where the laminae of the heel and bar attach to the collateral cartilage rather than bone, greater flexibility and movement is possible; however, it also makes them more susceptible to bending and collapse.

The ground surface of the bar needs to slope dorsally, up from the angle of the heel, to allow it to 'escape' from the descending pastern. As the bar is pushed down it can make greater ground contact to increase traction and

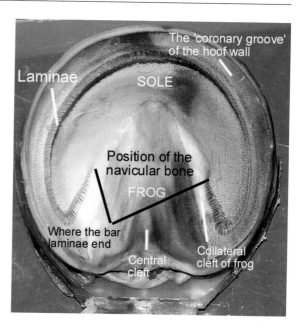

Fig. 106 ABOVE: *The two internal ridges of the empty hoof capsule are the collateral clefts (grooves) of the frog on a solar view of a foot. There is a dip on the internal ridges just anterior to the end of the laminae of the bars, which is where the navicular bone sits.*

Fig. 107 BELOW: *When weight is put on the leg, the fetlock and pastern bones drop. The distal end of P2 rotates on P3 in the coffin joint, and as it lowers, pushes between the collateral cartilages (CC). The descent of the navicular bone will be limited by the structures under it.*

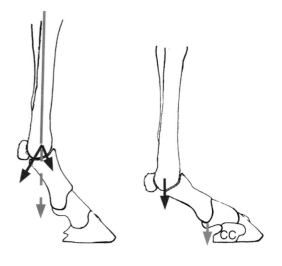

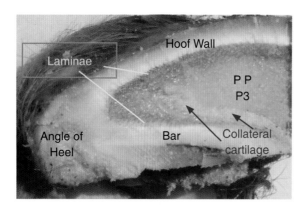

Fig. 108   Horizontal cut across a heel.

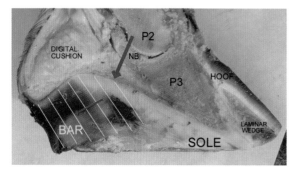

Fig. 109   A specimen from a horse with chronic laminitis, cut to expose the full extent of the bar. As weight is put on a foot, if the palmar edge of the bar is able to descend, a strong bar will push back on the angle of the heel to help keep it upright.

improve braking, but this movement of the bar will also provide support to the heel and help to maintain its angle. As weight is applied and the descending navicular bone pushes the anterior portion down towards the ground, the bar should rotate as a unit to act as a strut for the heel, pushing against the ground forces that might otherwise cause it to collapse. A weak bar that is bent will be less able to achieve this.

Bar Strength

The bar and the hoof horn of a horse will have similar strength, and the bars contribute to the shape of the strong- and weak-walled feet described in Chapter 4. Both the heels and bars remain straight and upright in feet with the strongest horn, with each part providing support for the other, whereas in those with the weakest horn, the bars buckle and collapse with the rest of the foot.

It is only the very strongest hooves that can maintain a heel angle the same as its dorsal wall, and most feet have a degree of in-turn of the heel and some curvature of the bar, these two features invariably occurring together. A heel that is not strong enough to withstand the forces on it will start to turn inwards and will take the posterior border of the bar with it, causing it to bend. The internal forces on a structurally weak, and now bent bar cause it to bend even more, thus further reducing its ability to support the heel.

Feet with only a small difference between hoof angle and heel angle have limited in-turn of the heel and bar, and are generally accepted as 'normal' because the bar is still effectively supporting the heel. For those with a greater difference of angle, the bars will have greater curvature, the heels will be more collapsed,

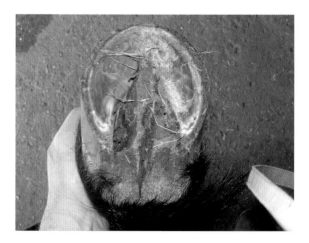

Fig. 110   A strong-walled hoof will have restricted heel expansion and will tend to have an upright foot and grow in an oval shape. The left fore of a Welsh pony.

and hoof function more likely to be impaired. The weakest feet have collapsed heels with a uniform curve to bars that grow almost horizontally over the sole. Sometimes there is an obvious, more localized fold in an area of the bar near to the heel, and this alters the way that the heel turns in.

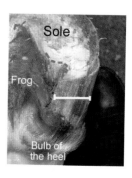

Fig. 112 A more localized fold in the bar accompanied by turn-in of only the most caudal (back) part of the heel.

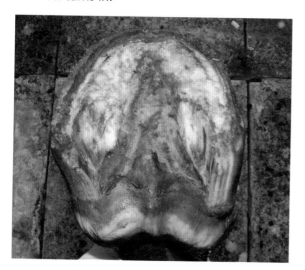

Fig. 111 The right forefoot of this Thoroughbred stallion has greater curvature of the lateral bar (on the left) and a straighter bar and more upright wall on the medial side.

- A curved bar that is growing over the adjoining sole in the collapsed foot
- The narrow upright foot with limited movement of the heels
- When splits appear at the bar/sole junction

The overgrowing, curved bar: The aim is to trim the bar (and heel) back to the more upright tubules and straighter form, to try to improve

Trimming the Bars

'Trim the bars if overgrown' seems to be the most common advice given on bar trimming, though there are some who suggest trimming more aggressively, while others say that they should never be touched. If too much bar is removed, their ability to support the internal structures and the heel will be reduced, but if left completely untrimmed they are likely to restrict foot function if strong, or become distorted if weak.

Any trimming of the bars must be to maintain or improve the support they provide, and to enhance heel movement, if this is restricted, to help absorb concussion. More aggressive bar trimming is indicated to rectify the following abnormalities:

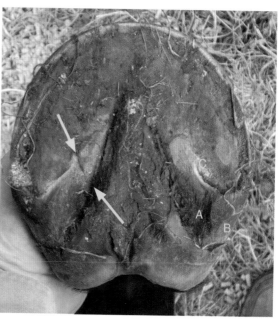

Fig. 113 Thoroughbred left forefoot. The medial bar (left) has a superficial crack at the level of the overlying navicular bone (between the yellow arrows). The lateral heel has a fold in the bar (A), turn-in of the back part of the heel (B), and a bar growing to cover the sole (C) (a superficial piece has been removed with a hoof knife).

support to the heel and take pressure off the sole in the seat of corn. Leaving these bars untrimmed, or trimming too much away, will both result in further heel collapse.

The narrow upright foot: The aim is to trim heel and bar to allow the restricted heels to move. The bars need to be trimmed to taper from the angles of the heel, to allow it to 'escape' from the descent of the navicular bone. In some circumstances, when heel height cannot be reduced – for example in some chronic laminitis cases and in club feet – greater trimming of the bar alone may be beneficial.

When splits appear at the bar/sole junction: The aim is to remove any distorted bar and the thickened sole on the two sides of the crack; this helps to even out the forces and prevent it from splitting further, when it would affect the sensitive dermis. A superficial crack at the junction of sole and bar is a fairly common feature of the overgrown bar, particularly in the weaker foot.

THE FROG

In Chapter 2, I described the position of the frog in relation to the other foot structures, and gave a few thoughts on what its function might be. The protection that it provides is not just a physical one, but also includes its ability to flex and adapt in order to compensate for uneven forces.

The Role of the Frog

The frog provides protection to internal structures above (dorsal to) it – to the deep digital flexor tendon, the navicular bone and navicular bursa; furthermore because it is flexible, it compensates for the movement of these parts as they absorb the increased weight put on the foot when the horse moves.

The frog also has a role in traction, since the greater the ground contact, the greater the friction between the frog and the ground.

Because it is a flexible structure, the frog allows more movement of the back part of the foot than if sole covered the whole of the bottom surface. It allows the two heels to move independently in both the median and transverse planes, helping the foot to compensate for uneven ground surfaces. This helps the foot to tolerate medio-lateral imbalance and uneven foot-landing – though if these are not corrected, over time they will lead to the foot becoming distorted with sheared or collapsed heels.

The frog has a role in hoof expansion and contraction, but this is more likely to be secondary to the physical separation of the collateral cartilages caused by the descent of P2 and the effect of pressure from the navicular bone on the bars, these being the primary factors.

The large numbers of sensory nerve endings in the frog transmit messages to the brain relating to the position of the foot (proprioception), identifying landing on uneven surfaces and allowing the horse to compensate. They also help to protect the frog and internal structures from damage by prompting the horse to evade external stimuli, by lifting the foot in response to sensory messages of pain. Horses can be completely sound without these sensory inputs, as demonstrated when investigating the cause of lameness with the use of nerve blocks (*see* Chapter 10), or when chronic painful foot conditions are managed by cutting the palmar digital nerves (neurectomy) – although in this case the foot becomes prone to damage because the horse is no longer aware of trauma to it, and will be less footsure on uneven ground.

Some of the forces of concussion and compression affecting the frog are absorbed as blood is forced through its venous plexus, and in the process, helps to pump venous blood and lymph back towards the heart.

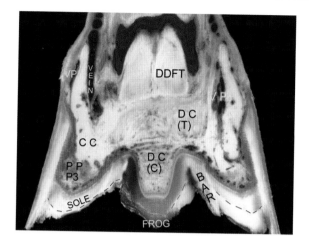
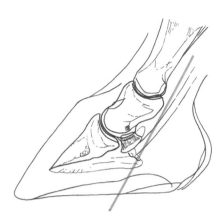

Figs. 114a and 114b   DDFT – deep digital flexor tendon. DC – digital cushion, (T) toric part, (C) cuneal part. CC – collateral cartilage. PP P3 – the palmar process of P3. VP and VP' are the deep and superficial venous plexuses.

The frog – the tan-coloured inner part (above the red broken line) – is hydrated, and outside this (below the line) is frog that has dried and hardened. The broken blue line identifies a similar demarcation in the sole. On the left, the outer layer (below the line) is dry and hard; on the right there is a greater depth of sole because more has been retained. It is only the superficial layer of this extra sole that has dried, and the deeper layers are able to stay hydrated. (Courtesy J-M Denoix, *The Equine Distal Limb*)

The ability of the frog to perform these functions relies on the 'correct' amount of ground contact. Too much contact is likely to cause bruising and discomfort, and not enough will reduce the effectiveness of frog function. Finding the correct balance is easier for the feral horse because their hoof length is controlled by the type of ground they live on. The feet of those living on soft ground will wear less and grow a longer hoof, but dirt can fill the space under the foot and provide ground contact to the frog, while abrasion of the hooves of those living in arid conditions means that the frog will be closer to the ground for it to make contact in these shorter feet. The frog is able to maintain an effective size in these situations by a balance between frog growth and the amount of wear; however, this is less likely to be the case for domesticated horses, particularly for those that are shod, but also for horses whose living and working surfaces are different.

Frog growth will be altered by factors that affect its blood supply. Blood flow through the foot increases with exercise but decreases

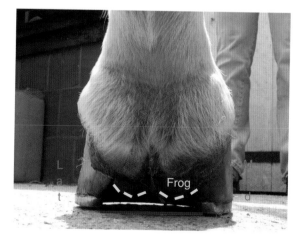

Figs. 115   In the shod foot, the frog may be some distance from the ground (blue line) when on a hard surface.

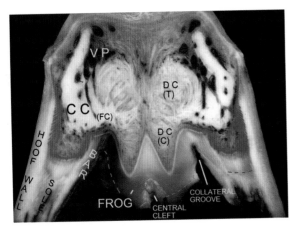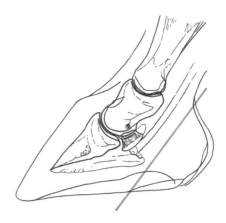

Figs. 116a and 116b   116 DC – digital cushion, (T) toric part and (C) the cuneal part. CC – collateral cartilage, with (FC) fibrocartilage on its inner (axial) surface. Near the back of the foot, the frog has a 'W' shape. Above the broken red line the frog is hydrated, and outside this line it has dried. The rest of the superficial layer must have been trimmed away before the specimen was produced. Above the broken blue line is hydrated sole (shown on the right of the picture). The sole is often thicker at the heel, because it tends to be retained in the space between the bar and the hoof wall. (Courtesy J-M Denoix The Equine Distal Limb)

in cold conditions, and blood circulation will improve with ground contact by the frog when the horse moves, but will be restricted if the frog is subjected to excessive pressure. The frog grows down from its corium in layers that are well attached, but provides weak points that allow it to shed rather than become overgrown (*see* Fig. 36).

The shape of the frog is derived from the form of the frog corium and how the frog grows out from this. The frog corium dips below the axial (inside) border of the sole in a 'U' shape (Fig. 114), and between the bars has a 'W' shape (Fig. 116), with the central sulcus (cleft) in the middle. Hooves that have limited expansion of the heels will maintain a compressed 'W' shape, which is why strong upright feet have a narrow frog with a deep central cleft, even when worked on a surface that provides ground contact with the frog. In feet that have developed with the more normal round shape, the 'W' will generally be flatter and the frog wider – although variation in shape doesn't necessarily coincide with the amount of ground contact. Thus a foot with

collapsed heels can have a narrow frog even though it has good ground contact.

As well as heel collapse, these cases often have substantial bars that are curved and are more horizontal than vertical (*see* Fig. 105) – so when the foot takes weight, there is inward movement of the heels and bars that counters any attempt made by the frog to expand.

Frog Trimming

Particularly in the unshod foot, when the hoof is trimmed the frog will probably also need to be trimmed to avoid leaving it prominent to the hoof wall, since excess pressure on the frog will cause bruising and discomfort. Other than this situation, whether to trim and what to trim becomes less well defined. The aim has to be to enable the frog to fulfil its functions, which will depend on whether the horse is shod, and the surface that the horse works on. Most people will remove any ragged edges, since they are remnants of a partially shed layer

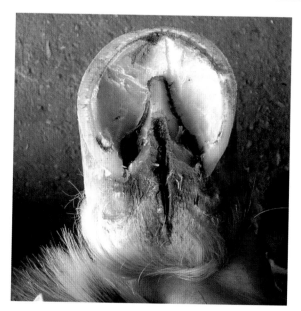

Fig. 117   In the strong upright foot, restriction of heel expansion will limit the spread of the frog, which remains narrow, with a deep central cleft.

structures that predispose them to pathological problems. Dirt that collects under the foot and fills the spaces benefits the horse by reducing peripheral loading. If this dirt benefits foot function, the question is whether we should leave this in place, or regularly pick out the feet? The requirement to do so is probably greater for horses kept in our environment, in the UK, than it may be elsewhere. With our wet conditions for much of the year, removal of mud and dirt gives the horn structures of the foot an opportunity to dry and harden. Also, picking out the clefts will remove flints or other sharp

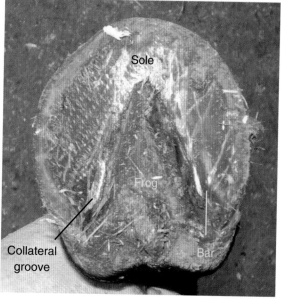

Fig. 118   A well proportioned foot with a healthy functional frog (the right fore of a Thoroughbred yearling).

and are unlikely to have much beneficial effect on frog function; moreover leaving them may provide sites for bacteria to multiply and thrush to develop.

In Fig. 114, hydrated flexible frog can be seen as the light brown covering to the frog dermis, and external to this is a lighter-coloured layer that is dehydrated and harder. In Fig. 116, the frog has obviously been trimmed prior to the dissection and a lot of this protective layer has been removed. The harder outer surface of the frog gives better protection from external trauma, and reduces the discomfort caused by localized pressure on the frog dermis from stones and uneven ground, so is generally better left untrimmed. If it is removed, in dry conditions the next layer will quickly harden, but until it does so, and in wet conditions, the frog will be more sensitive to stony and uneven ground.

Constant peripheral loading of a foot, as can occur when shod, results in changes to internal

stones picked up in the field, as well as faeces and soiled bedding from the stable, all of which can potentially cause damage to the frog and other horn structures.

Horses turned out all the time, and those stabled on very clean beds will, in most cases, have no problem if the feet are not picked out, but those constantly stood in mud or

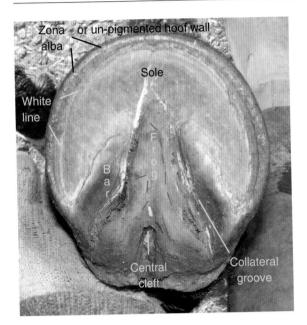

Fig. 119   *The left fore of a pony kept on pasture (in February in wet conditions). The whole of the previous sole layer has been shed, leaving the sole completely smooth. The relatively smooth surface of the frog has lines on it with slight fraying (broken red lines): these are the edges of different frog layers, where the pieces or layers will separate.*

in soiled bedding will be more prone to infection. In any case, the feet should still be checked regularly.

THE SOLE

To examine the sole thoroughly, it needs to be picked out and washed with water.

Concavity of the sole is a desirable feature, whereas a 'flat foot' is not. Part of the foot's anti-concussion mechanism is the ability of the sole to drop when weight is put on the foot, allowing the hoof wall to flex, and in some circumstances, to improve traction by 'cupping' on softer ground. The ability of the foot to do this is reduced in a foot with a flattened sole. Sole concavity is best assessed once the foot has been trimmed.

Movement of the sole, or lack of it, in response to thumb pressure can give an idea of sole thickness, but will depend on the sole's moisture content, having greater pliability in wet conditions and reduced flexibility if dry. Features on the underside of the foot allow estimation of sole thickness, with the depth of the collateral clefts (grooves) on each side of the frog being a good indicator, since the thickness of the frog commissures, where it attaches to the sole at the base of the clefts, is relatively constant. This distance is about 1cm, which is the depth that the dermis of the sole and frog are able to keep hydrated (Figs 114 and 116).

If the rest of the sole were the same depth as at the commissures, it would be insufficient to give adequate protection and comfort, but this is provided by the addition of more layers, and dehydration and hardening of the superficial layer. The depth of the collateral grooves between the frog and sole therefore tells us the depth of these additional layers of sole – the greater the thickness, the greater the protection to the underlying dermis.

If the surface of the sole is cracked, this generally indicates a thicker sole. In feet where loss of sole from abrasion is limited, it is generally prevented from becoming too thick by its ability to shed layers. The outer layer dries out and hardens to help protect from injury, though having dried, this hard 'crust' becomes liable to cracking. Cracking allows air to get to the layer below, which then starts to lose moisture and to harden prior to the loss of the superficial protecting layer. The cracked sole generally breaks away in pieces, or may be cleaned away by the farrier or trimmer. In dry conditions, the attachment between the layers degenerates, and this is the white powdery material on the surface of the piece removed (Fig. 121).

There may be prominent areas on the sole, most commonly where sole is retained alongside the frog. Because it is fused with the end of the bar, it appears as an extension to the

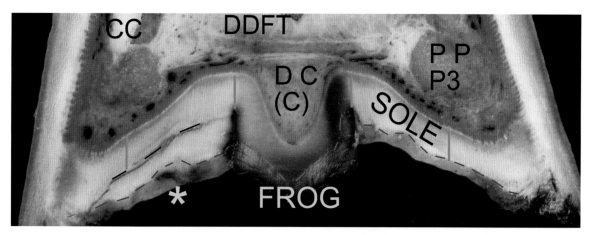

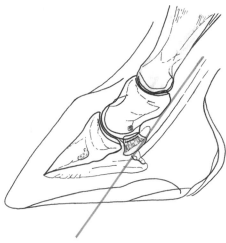

Figs. 120 and 120a   DDFT – deep digital flexor tendon, DC (C) – digital cushion (cuneal part), CC – collateral cartilage, PP P3 – palmar process of P3. Uniform thickness of a hydrated sole, frog, and the commissures of the frog (green lines). Below the broken red line on the frog and the broken blue line on the sole is the outer, dehydrated layer. This is deeper at the yellow * where there is a crack in the outer layer. On the left side of the image, the sole is thicker because sole layers have not been shed. The broken black line is where a fissure has developed, which would have been followed by the shedding of all the layers below this. **(Courtesy J-M Denoix *The Equine Distal Limb*)**

bar and is sometimes referred to as such, but it is derived from solar corium. Examples of this can be seen in a number of photographs earlier in the chapter, and in Fig. 36, the sole next to the frog can be seen to have retained layers of sole. In some cases, the raised area of sole may even extend as a prominent ridge to completely surround the frog. Some people suggest that this raised area of sole is the result of stimulated growth in response to external factors, in a similar way that in man, repeated pressure rubbing on the skin of prominent parts of the hand or foot causes callus formation. If this were the case for the horse's sole, then it would be expected that those exercised more would have larger sole callus; however the opposite is generally the case.

Rather than sole thickening in this area being due to extra growth, it appears to be due to delayed shedding (Figs 120 and 122), being seen most frequently in strong-walled feet that have less flexibility. Sometimes bruising can be seen in the sole after it has been removed, but this will be as a result of, rather than the cause of, the prominent sole. Opinions differ on whether this sole ridge should be removed or not. Those who believe it to be extra sole that has formed to provide more protection will leave it in place, while others do so because they know that if a foot is trimmed correctly and the horse is exercised, it will be shed. If a horse is worked on hard and uneven surfaces with these ridges left in place, sole bruising can occur under them.

Figs. 121 and 121a   Cracking of the retained hardened sole of a Thoroughbred (stabled due to injury). The attachment between layers tends to become white and crumbly when it dries out, as seen on the underside of the piece of sole (inset).

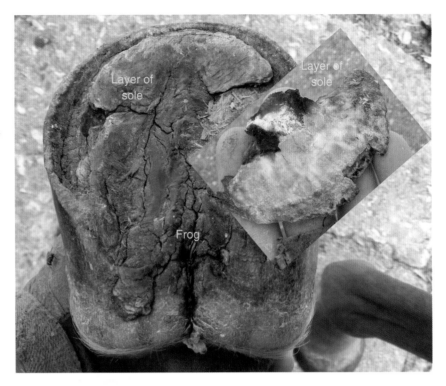

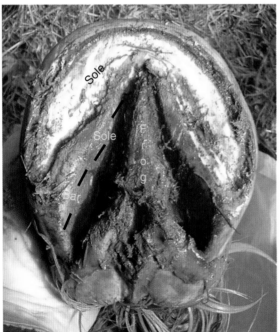

Fig. 122   Fore foot of a Welsh Cob (a strong foot, as can be seen from the straightness of the bars) with retained sole, kept at pasture but not exercised. This was also seen in the hind feet at the same time.

'Distal descent of P3' is a term sometimes used to describe the downward (distal) displacement of P3 relative to the hoof capsule as a result of reduced support for the bone. The most obvious situation for P3 to lose its support is following laminitis, when it is more commonly described as 'rotation' or 'sinking' (*see* Chapter 7), but can occur when the laminae are intact simply from flaring of the hoof wall. The stability the wall and white line give to the outer rim of the sole helps to support P3 all around the foot by providing a 'ledge' for the edge of the bone to rest on. If the wall flares this support moves away, leaving the edge of the bone resting on more flexible sole, which allows P3 to descend distally and may be evident on the sole as a prominent ridge running around inside the 'white line' (Figs 123 and 124).

This prominent rim of sole is sometimes referred to as 'sole callous', but it is no thicker than the adjacent sole. Removing any of this prominent sole is likely to weaken it and compound the problem by further reducing

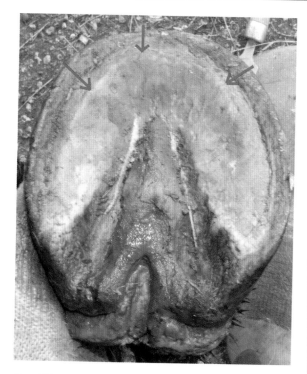

Fig. 123 *Foot of a pregnant Thoroughbred mare kept at pasture, in wet conditions. The solar border of P3 has caused a slight prominence of the sole inside its junction with the 'white line'.*

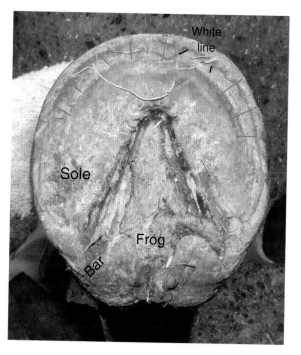

P3 support, so it is important that it is left untouched and steps taken to address the underlying cause, in this case the flaring of the hoof wall.

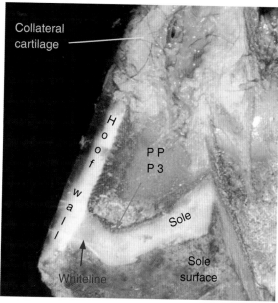

Fig. 125 *The frog removed (the right edge of the picture) and the heel sliced off a cadaver specimen of a Thoroughbred foot. PP P3 – palmar process of P3. The hoof wall and 'white line' have moved outwards, and the solar border of P3 is resting on unsupported sole (red arrow), resulting in the sort of change seen in Fig. 124.*

Sole Thickness

In most situations sole thickness is 'self-maintained' by the horse, with increasing rate of growth in response to stimulus, or by shedding a layer if sole is not lost from abrasion. There are some situations where this balance is affected and the horse is sore from thin soles or has discomfort from reduced hoof function from retained sole.

Fig. 124 *Thoroughbred foot with a more marked distal descent of P3, with a prominent sole and recessed 'white line' (between the wall and sole, and covered by dirt in the image).*

There have been a number of studies measuring the feet of domestic and feral horses, which have included measuring sole thickness. Sole thickness seems to vary, to some extent, between breeds, but also horses of the same breed in different environments can have differences in sole thickness. Sole thickness under the tip of P3 is most commonly between 10–15mm, and considered thin if less than this. Soles much thicker than 15mm generally have retained sole, and may be even thicker if a horse is regularly shod with pads. Sole is generally thicker around its perimeter (*see* Figs 114 and 120) and also in the back half of the foot, where sole is retained between the bar and wall (*see* Fig. 116).

What happens to retained sole depends on whether conditions are wet or dry. In dry conditions, the dry superficial layer cracks and breaks away. In wet conditions the superficial layer remains pliable, and because it doesn't crack, the connection between it and the layer above doesn't get the opportunity to dry out, so the outer layer stays attached. Because a wet sole stays flexible, it doesn't give so much protection to its sensitive dermis from stones and uneven ground, and thickening of the sole helps it to do so. When ground conditions change and these feet are able to dry out, the superficial layer hardens, cracks, and then breaks away as normal.

If thick soles stay wet, the sole material does degenerate, and when the farrier or trimmer attends to the foot, crumbly sole can be scraped away easily. This crumbly material loses any pigment when it degenerates, and unless dirt penetrates, is always white, as seen in the thin line produced by my hoof knife in the soft pigmented sole in Fig. 119.

Thin Soles

Loss of sole from trauma, trimming or excessive wear produces thinner soles which may affect soundness, and thinning of the sole is seen in cases of laminitis, where pressure is increased locally under the tip of P3. In these cases, the real problem arises when this is combined with increased external pressure, with the dropped sole pressing either on the ground or some form of 'sole support' which has been applied to the foot.

The environment and the way we manage horses will have an effect on the thickness of the sole and the protection it provides. A horse will very likely become footsore if kept in a muddy field and then worked on a hard, abrasive surface. When we initially discard our shoes and socks on a beach holiday, our soles are sensitive and we have to walk carefully on all but soft and stone-free sand – but by the end of the holiday we can cope far better. The surface of the sole hardens, with dirt becoming embedded in the surface, and thickens by reduction of sole shedding. People who live without shoes in dry environments develop a hard leathery

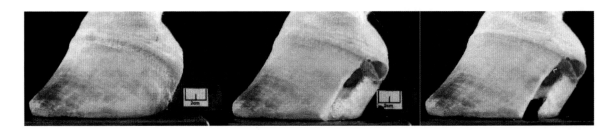

Fig. 126 *This specimen was dissected by Mike Savoldi, initially removing a section from the heel to expose the great depth of sole. In the third picture he has removed the crumbly, drier sole to leave only the deep layer of hydrated sole. (Images courtesy Mike Savoldi)*

sole that allows them to cope with virtually any terrain. This seems to be the same situation for feral horses in the USA (mustangs) and Australia (brumbies): these have been found to have a good thickness (about 15mm) of hard sole that allows them to travel great distances over hard terrain.

Providing similar circumstances to allow 'conditioning' of the soles of horses in the UK can be extremely difficult to achieve due to our wet conditions through the autumn and winter (and beyond), and it is because of this that the majority of working horses in the UK are shod. It takes greater effort and commitment to manage a working horse unshod in these conditions – although there are sufficient examples of them around to show that it is achievable. In some cases this is only made possible by working the horse in hoof boots.

Thick Soles

When too much sole is retained, it can become thick enough to limit sole and hoof movement, something that is sometimes referred to as being 'sole bound'. Long-term use of pads under shoes can do this if excess sole is not removed each time the horse is re-shod. Some claims are made about the effectiveness of applying 'this' or 'that' shoe, cast or boot on a horse to increase sole thickness. In many cases, it probably achieves this more from sole retention than any increase in sole growth from 'improved circulation' as claimed.

Becoming sole bound is really only a problem of the horse with a strong hoof wall because the flexibility of weaker walls is more likely to let retained sole crack and loosen, for it to be shed. Strong feet that are upright (tall heels) will have very thick sole between the wall and the bar, and this will limit the movement of the heels; however, this is probably the result of the rigidity of these structures rather than the cause of it, but if this thick sole is left in place it will only compound the problem.

7 Laminitis

Laminitis is an extremely serious disease which can affect the feet of any equid but is, in reality, a problem of the domesticated horse, pony and donkey. It is a painful condition occurring as a result of the separation of the laminae with the loss of support of the bone inside the hoof. It is very common and, unfortunately, is becoming more so, and if horse owners reading this have not had experience of it, they will almost certainly know someone who has.

Over the past thirty years my explanation of laminitis to clients has changed significantly, as well as frequently, as new theories have been put forward and the old ones discarded. Extensive research has provided a lot more information about laminitis, but sadly this has still not produced answers to many questions, and a lot of the advice given is still confusing and even contradictory.

SYMPTOMS OF LAMINITIS

The period after the initiating cause, before any clinical symptoms of laminitis are seen, is referred to as the developmental stage. When

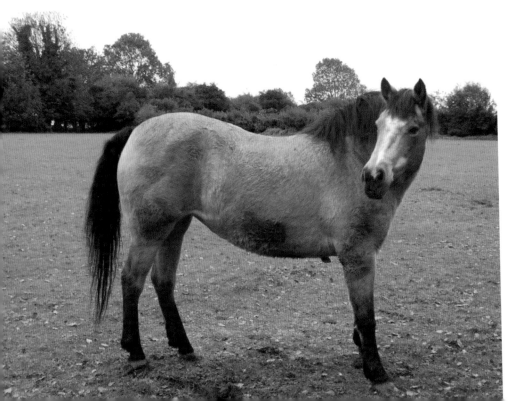

Fig. 127 Pony with chronic laminitis suffering another acute episode of laminitis, placing the fore feet out in front to try to reduce the pain.

caused experimentally, we know this phase is around thirty hours when the trigger is a carbohydrate (for example, grain) overload or insulin-induced (*see* Chapter 8). Black walnut extract (BWE) is sometimes used to induce laminitis experimentally, but is unusual, taking only around ten hours before symptoms are seen (*see* Laminitis Triggers, below). Although no symptoms are evident until these times, *changes in the laminae start to occur much earlier than this.*

Acute Laminitis

The symptoms of acute laminitis include lameness and difficulty turning and, when standing, the horse may change its stance and shift its weight between limbs. The other very common symptom is an increase in the strength of the digital pulse.

Initially there are no visible hoof changes in first-time acute laminitis, however, in more severe cases, where there is extensive separation, rotation of P3 can leave a palpable

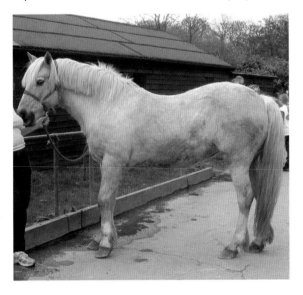

Fig. 128 Weight-shifting is most obvious when the front feet are affected. The pony lifts one foot and then the other.

hollow in the skin at the top of the hoof, where the coronary band has been pulled down with the bone. In the most severe cases, when all the laminae are damaged, the coronary dip can extend all round the foot (a 'sinker').

The greater the separation that occurs in the acute stage, the longer and more difficult it is for the horse to recover, so it is very important that laminitis cases are treated as soon as possible, to limit the damage.

Sometimes mild cases of laminitis are difficult to differentiate from other foot conditions, but if there is any chance, from clinical signs, that a horse could have laminitis, it should always be treated as such.

Weight shifting: The horse may shift its weight from one limb to another, sometimes lifting the relieved foot off the ground. This is more obvious when it occurs in the front feet, where this sort of behaviour is very unusual, whereas hind feet are often rested in normal circumstances.

Change in stance: The stance will vary, depending on which feet, and how many of them, are affected. In milder cases there may be no change from the normal stance. If more painful, the horse will often stand with its fore feet placed out in front, in an attempt to reduce the pressure on its painful toes (Fig. 127); in more severe cases this may be accompanied by the hind feet being positioned forward under the body to bear more of the weight. This would be considered to be the 'classic' laminitis stance.

Lameness: This usually involves more than one foot, and more commonly affects the front feet; however, it can involve only one foot, or up to all four feet, and in any combination. The degree of lameness will depend on the severity of the laminitis attack, which the

Swedish scientist Obel was able to demonstrate over sixty years ago. Obel used four lameness descriptions to grade the severity of laminitis, when he found that there was a close correlation between the amount of separation seen histologically (under the microscope) and the severity of the lameness exhibited. These grades are: lame only at trot; lame at walk but willing to do so; very lame and reluctant to move; cannot be moved, and if down, difficult to make stand up – and Obel's grades one to four are still used today to describe the severity of lameness.

As the level of pain increases, the posterior phase of the stride becomes shortened, as the horse tries to avoid putting pressure on the toe. When very sore, the front foot stride is even more limited, with the horse keeping its feet out in front and greater weight taken on the hind legs. The hind feet may show an exaggerated lift at walk if they are more painful than the fore feet.

Difficulty turning: The horse finds it difficult to turn and does so with a shuffling motion, with the front feet placed out in front of it.

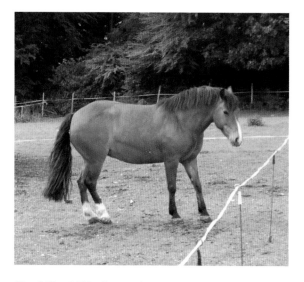

Fig. 129   Difficulty turning in acute laminitis (in an insulin-resistant pony).

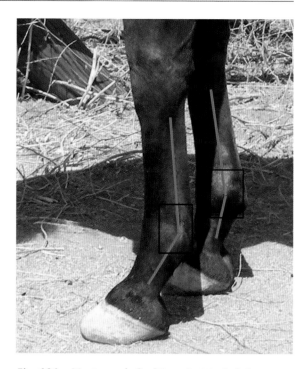

Fig. 130   Most people find it easiest to feel the 'digital pulse' in the digital arteries as they pass over the sesamoid bones (the black boxes on the image) on both sides of the leg; the lateral site is shown on the left fore and the medial site on the right fore.

Increased digital pulse: An increase in the force of the pulse of the digital arteries occurs with acute laminitis – although this can also accompany severe bruising of the sole or an abscess. An obvious digital pulse in more than one foot is likely to occur only with laminitis.

Heat in the foot: Heat may be felt in the coronary band or hoof, but again, this is not specific for laminitis and occurs with other foot conditions, or can just be due to environmental conditions or exercise.

Sub-acute Laminitis

Sub-acute laminitis refers to the stage after the acute phase when the cause of the laminitis has been controlled; depending on the extent of the damage and how the horse is managed, it either leads to healing and resolution, or progresses to a chronic state.

Chronic Laminitis

'Chronic' may be used to describe cases that are slow to respond, or when laminitis recurs, but the common feature is some degree of displacement of P3 inside the hooves.

When the bone and hoof separate, the normally balanced forces in the foot change, and the hoof loses its stability and deforms. This alters the blood flow to different parts of the foot, which causes differential rates of hoof growth around the foot. Chronic laminitis cases can show any of the signs described for acute laminitis, but will also have visible changes in the feet.

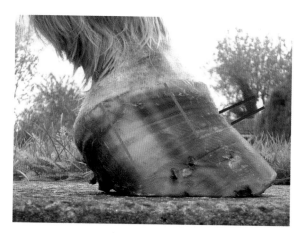

Fig. 131   Chronic laminitis: commonly there are changes in the line of the dorsal wall (two sites – the blue lines) and divergence of the growth rings around the hoof (faster growth at the heels than at the toe – the red lines).

Foot Changes in Chronic Laminitis

In chronic laminitis there is a change in the line of the dorsal wall, and there may be more than

one change in angle, depending on how many bouts of laminitis have occurred within the growth period of the wall (*see* Fig. 131).

If the deviated dorsal wall is rasped back

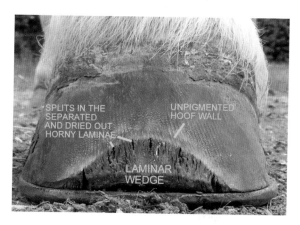

Fig. 132   The front foot of a chronic laminitic pony. The separated dorsal wall was rasped back in line with the new growth at the top of the wall when it was last shod. The rasping exposed unpigmented hoof, separated laminae and laminar wedge. At this stage, these areas have dried and are now hard.

Fig. 133   The horn produced by the damaged and distorted terminal papillae makes the 'white line' wider and weaker than normal, and splits develop that allow the entry of dirt to set up abscesses. SC = solar cavity that has occurred between layers of sole.

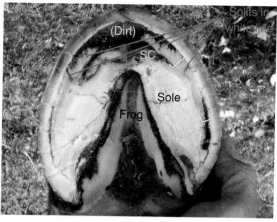

in line with the new growth at the top of the wall, separated laminae may be seen, as in Fig.

132. In acute laminitis, the space left when the laminae separate is filled with fluid, but in chronic laminitis this has become filled with disorganized keratinous material referred to as 'laminar' or 'lamellar wedge'.

The feet commonly have obvious hoof rings, with indentations, and the distance between these is often wider at the heels than on the dorsal wall. This is generally considered to be due to slower growth of the dorsal wall because of pressure on the coronary blood supply. Continuing differences in the rate of growth indicate that uneven forces persist!

The white line is wider and of poor quality, and splits are often present. Sometimes pink discolouration is visible on the sole in a crescent in front of the frog. This is seen about six weeks after a laminitis episode, which is the time it takes for sole changes occurring in a laminitis episode to grow out (*see* Fig. 134). In more severe cases, the sole may become convex under P3 and drop below the level of the hoof wall. There is a danger that the tip of P3 will penetrate the sole in this situation (*see* Fig. 146).

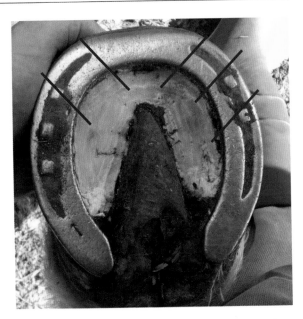

Fig. 134 Crescent area of discoloration on the sole (blue lines) seven weeks after an undiagnosed mild lameness. The fore foot of a Welsh cob.

LAMINITIS TRIGGERS

Because the 'cause of laminitis' is often used to refer to the mechanisms inside the foot that bring about separation of the laminae as well as the factors that initiate these changes, I will try to differentiate between them by using 'cause' for what produces the changes in the feet and 'trigger' for what sets them off.

The vast majority of laminitis cases occur as a result of disease processes happening elsewhere in the body, and laminitis can be considered as a symptom of these conditions. Other than the effect of mechanical forces directly on the feet, the triggers of laminitis follow metabolic and hormonal disturbances, and/or infectious and inflammatory conditions:

Mechanical separation – 'road founder' – can occur following fast or prolonged work. Mechanical damage may be a cause of laminitis in racing Thoroughbreds with hooves that have spread and flared, leaving P3 less well supported. It may be more insidious, to cause the changes found in the feet of Brumbies living in arid conditions in Australia, which have to travel great distances for food and water.

'Dependent-leg laminitis' can occur in a foot constantly taking weight when the opposite leg is badly injured and not weight-bearing.

Metabolic and hormonal disturbances: Equine metabolic syndrome (EMS) refers to the systemic changes accompanying insulin resistance, which includes laminitis as a symptom. The role of insulin resistance (IR) is discussed at length in Chapter 8.

Laminitis is also a symptom of PPID ('pituitary pars intermedia disease', or Cushing's disease), *see* Chapter 8.

Laminitis may follow the administration of corticosteroids (*see* Chapter 8).

Inflammatory and infectious conditions:
An excessive intake of carbohydrates, commonly referred to as 'carbohydrate overload' (CHO), causes disturbance in the gut flora of the caecum and large intestine, and can result in laminitis. CHO comes from ingesting the starch in grain – either from raiding the feed bins or directly from over-feeding – and the fructans in pasture (oligofructose is used to experimentally induce laminitis). 'Pasture-related laminitis' is discussed in Chapter 8. Similar changes occur in the gut following an acute intestinal condition such as colic or colitis.

Laminitis can be triggered by infection: typically this accompanies metritis following a retained placenta, but it can follow pneumonia or abscesses.

Laminitis may also occur with specific diseases: for example occurring commonly with Potomac fever as a result of colitis, which is a common symptom of the disease. There is also a suggested association with Lyme's disease.

Black walnut wood shavings, when used in error as stable bedding, can cause laminitis. (Black walnut extract – BWE – is used experimentally to induce laminitis.)

Stress – systemic, metabolic or psychological – may also trigger laminitis (by affecting cortisol production and affecting IR): *see* Chapter 8.

FOOT CHANGES IN LAMINITIS

In laminitis, the attachment between the hoof (horny laminae) and the dermis (sensitive laminae) is damaged and they separate, with the site of separation, whatever the cause, being at the level of the basement membrane. Damage to the basement membrane, or the connections of the horny laminae to it, reduces the ability of the laminae to hold P3 in position.

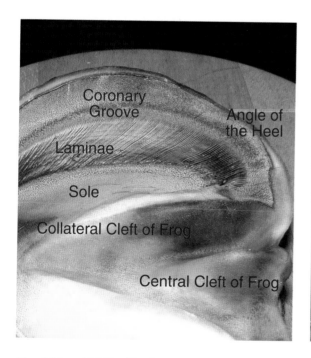

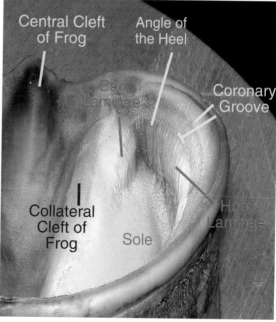

Figs. 135 and 135b   The 'horny' laminae extend round to the angle of the heel and then forward for the bar. The internal ridges are the clefts of the frog when looked at from underneath the foot.

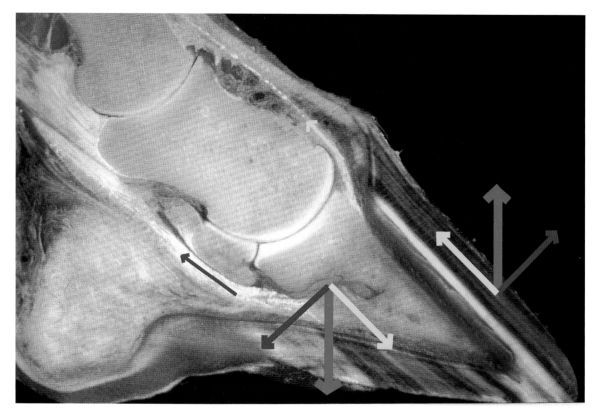

Fig. 136   The red arrows depict the weight of the horse and the opposing ground-reaction force. The yellow vector is of greater significance when the horse is standing, and the blue arrows come more into play when the horse moves (same parasagittal cut as in Fig. 37) (Image courtesy J-M. Denoix, **The Equine Distal Limb***).*

Since laminitis is generally a consequence of systemic changes, all the laminae are potentially affected, as is the basement membrane attachment to the coronary corium, the frog corium, the sole corium and the terminal papillae.

The reason there is laminar separation in some parts of the foot and not in others appears to be due to the difference in mechanical forces acting on them. Whatever the cause of the separation, the same mechanical forces apply and there is a consistent pattern of separation in the foot. This always starts in the front of the foot, down the dorsal wall, indicating that this is where the greatest mechanical forces are exerted on the laminae.

The forces acting on the laminae are from

P3 (the weight of the horse and the pull of the extensor and flexor tendons on the bone), and the ground-reaction forces on the hoof. The force from the digital extensor comes from the branch of the suspensory ligament that crosses the pastern and attaches to it (Fig. 16b c').

Separation is brought about by forces causing the bone to move away from the hoof wall, but also involves the hoof wall being pulled away from the bone. Whether it is the horse's weight or the effect of the deep flexor tendon on P3, following the loss of the attachment at the dorsal wall, the bone rotates so that its tip presses on to the sole.

The stretching and separation of the laminae, and the pressure of the tip of the bone on to

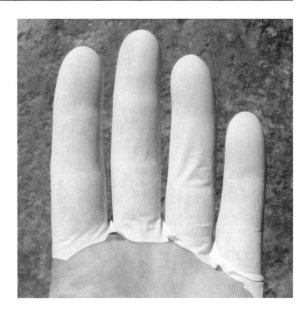

Fig. 137   Imagination required! The hand represents the primary lamella and the fingers the secondary lamellae, with the fingers of a rubber glove covering them representing the basement membrane. Pulling on the glove at the tips of the fingers initially leaves a space at the tips but the glove fingers stay in place. This is what occurs with the basement membrane and the secondary lamellae with Grade I damage. As more force is applied, the glove fingers start to slip off the fingers, which is what occurs with the basement membrane in Grade II laminitis. The secondary lamellae are flexible structures (unlike fingers) so, as more force is applied, these become stretched as the basement membrane is pulled away. Grade III laminitis will have further lengthening of the secondary lamellae and further detachment of the basement membrane. In Grade IV laminitis, the 'fingers' of the glove will have completely slipped off the fingers. (Try this.)

the solar corium, seem to be the sources of pain in the acute case.

Studies on experimentally induced acute laminitis have demonstrated that there is a good correlation between the amount of pain shown by the horse and the degree of separation of the laminae.

If damage continues to the extent that all the laminae separate, there is nothing to hold the bone in place and P3 sinks inside the hoof (referred to as a 'sinker').

Pathogenesis of Laminitis

There is still great debate about what actually occurs in the feet to cause separation of the laminae in laminitis (pathogenesis). The short-list includes the following:
- Inflammation (and oedema)
- Vascular – disruption of the blood supply
- Enzyme activation
- Altered glucose metabolism
- Mechanical separation

Many other causes have also been suggested.

Research, in the past, generally studied animals that were already showing symptoms of laminitis, but even though modern research on experimentally induced laminitis is helping to identify what occurs early in the developmental stage of laminitis, we still do not know whether some of the changes that have been identified have a primary role or are a consequence of laminitis. However, it does appear that different mechanisms can cause laminitis in different situations, and that often there will be a combination of triggers involved.

My (Current) Opinion on Pathogenesis

Mechanical separation: Although likely to be rarely the single causative factor in laminitis, the mechanical forces on the bone and the hoof will affect how much separation occurs, in every case of laminitis, whatever the cause.

A change in glucose metabolism of the basal cells: This has been proposed as the trigger in metabolic causes of laminitis (*see* Chapter 8). Altered glucose metabolism (IR) is likely to be an underlying problem in most cases of pasture-related laminitis, but is also likely to have some involvement in other laminitis cases caused by other triggers. Even if not contributing to laminitis developing, the effect of stress, lack of exercise and, in some cases, an inappropriate diet once laminitis has occurred, may result in IR becoming a factor in the ongoing progression of the laminitis.

Inflammation: Occurs only in some forms of laminitis, and now appears to be as an immediate response to damage from whatever triggers laminar separation, rather than being the cause of the separation. When the trigger has passed, or has been removed, inflammation is no longer a factor in laminar separation.

Vascular changes: There is fairly strong evidence that changes to the laminar blood supply play a part in laminitis, but rather than the theory that laminitis is caused by reduced capillary blood flow due to blood being diverted through the arterio-venous (A-V) shunts, it is more likely that they are due to the effect of IR and/or endogenous (the horse's own) corticosteroids on the blood vessels.

Enzyme (MMP) activation: Seems to be a factor in the extensive laminar separation occurring in carbohydrate overload, colic, colitis and Potomac fever, and also with metritis and other infections; however, there is now doubt that this is the initiating cause in laminitis. MMP activation is not a feature of insulin-induced laminitis.

There appears, both clinically and from histology, that there are two mechanisms involved in laminar separation; from the loss of integrity of the epidermal basal cell layer, and from disruption of the basement membrane and its attachment to the basal cells due to increased MMP activity. In some cases, both of these occur at the same time, and since inflammation and impaired blood flow seem

to have a role in causing them, and it is the mechanical forces on the bone and hoof which pull the laminae apart, it is not surprising that there is still so much confusion about the pathophysiology and pathogenesis of laminitis. (For further comment on pathogenesis, *see* Chapter 12.)

FIRST AID

When symptoms of laminitis become evident, separation of the laminae has already started. Action should be taken immediately to limit the damage.

- Contact your vet: your vet can only give advice and attend your horse promptly, to start treatment, if they know there is a problem, so contact them.
- Provide support to the sole or frog.
- Try to work out what the laminitis triggers might be, and immediately take steps to remove or control them.

Frog and Sole Support

With the hoof wall and the bone starting to move in opposite directions, it is important to provide support under the foot since this reduces peripheral loading on the hoof wall and helps to stabilize the internal structures of the foot. This is generally achieved by the application of something underneath the foot, but standing the horse on a firm but conforming surface will help.

It is important that external pressure is not applied under the tip of an unstable bone, so a 'frog support', or conforming material covering the back half of the foot is safest in the chronic laminitic, and this will often give an immediate improvement in comfort. It is for fear of pressure damage to the sole and tip of P3 that some people advise against any use of

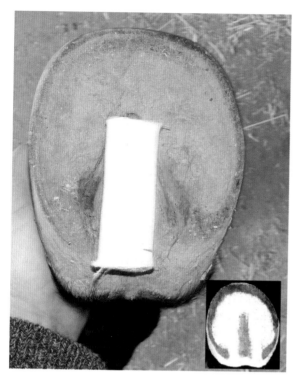

Fig. 138 *A 'Frog support' can be something as simple as a bandage taped over the frog.*

from pasture, having been found lame in the field – although moving a horse with acute laminitis can cause further separation of the laminae. It should be safe enough to walk the horse a short distance if it is happy to do so, and provided support has been taped to the bottom of the foot. If the horse is reluctant to walk or it is some distance from the stable, it is best to leave it where it is to await the arrival of the vet, and arrangements should be put in place to transport the horse back to a stable.

TREATMENT

> *André Previn:* You are playing all the wrong notes.
> *Eric Morecambe:* I am playing all the right notes [pause], but not necessarily in the right order.
> *Morecambe and Wise Christmas Special*
> (TV) 1971

Doing the right thing at the wrong time seems to be a particular problem when it comes to treating laminitis, partly because of the conflicting information available. It is difficult for an owner or stable manager to know if they should apply ice or heat to the feet, provide strict rest or allow movement or even force a horse to walk, apply sole support or frog support, have the feet trimmed with low heels or the foot left tilted, have the heels wedged up after trimming or the foot left flat, or whether the horse should be shod (and the type of shoe) or left unshod (booted or unbooted).

All these options have been proposed as methods of treatment for cases of laminitis – and most of them still are – and it is possible that there are circumstances when each option is the best one. An owner must also decide whether to allow the horse access to grass or not, and if not, then what alternative to use (hay or haylage), as well as what medication and which supplement might or might not be suitable.

full 'sole support', but in acute laminitis cases it should be completely safe, and actually the best option. It is important to understand that the role of these is not to directly support the bone, but to assist the solar structures to do so.

There are several materials that are commonly used by vets and farriers as frog or sole supports, such as Styrofoam or EVA (ethyl vinyl acetate) blocks, pads or dental impression material, but as a first aid measure, strapping any compressible pad, or even a bag of sand, under the foot or taping a small bandage or Lilypad under the frog will generally be adequate, and safe, in the short term. Obviously a greater thickness of material will be required if the horse is shod.

It is essential to *remove the cause of the laminitis, or move the horse from the cause.* This will most commonly involve removing the horse

Treatment must involve controlling any trigger factor, giving treatment for the cause of laminitis, reducing the forces causing separation, and dealing with the individual circumstances in any given case.

Treating the Laminitis Trigger

Until the trigger is controlled, separation is liable to continue. Some of the more acute and severe cases of laminitis are likely to occur in a veterinary hospital situation, where the horse has been admitted for a colic operation or colitis, and treatment for these has already been started, which may include the application of cryotherapy (ice treatment) to at-risk cases. Similar situations may occur in the field, where antibiotics can be given for infections, NSAIDs (flunixin or ketoprofen) for endotoxaemia, and fluid therapy for systemic and toxaemic conditions.

Other situations will involve removing the horse from the cause, which in many cases will be taking a horse off grass. In some situations the trigger will already have passed, but laminitis cases triggered by metabolic or hormonal changes need these problems to be addressed, otherwise the trigger will be ongoing (*see* Chapter 8).

Treating the Cause of the Laminar Separation

The fact that people talk about what they believe causes laminitis and then proceed to medicate for all the other possible causes as well is actually understandable since, as was pointed out earlier, there will often be multiple factors involved at the same time, either with primary or secondary roles.

A huge range of drugs has been used to treat laminitis, and their use has been based on whatever the current theory on pathogenesis

> MEDICINES AND SUPPLEMENTS PROVEN TO PREVENT THE DEVELOPMENT OF LAMINITIS OR TO STOP ITS PROGRESS:
>
> NONE!

was popular at that time, but sadly there is none that has been proven to prevent laminitis or to limit the progress of the disease. The problem is that treating laminitis is like dealing with a biting dog, because you don't know whether something is working or not until you are 'bitten again', and only then do you know that it hasn't.

Medication for Inflammation and Pain Relief

Non-steroidal anti-inflammatory drugs (NSAIDs) – most commonly phenylbutazone ('bute') and flunixin (Finadyne/Banamine) – are the most common group of drugs used in the treatment of laminitis, and as well as being anti-inflammatory they are also analgesic (painkillers).

I have already expressed my doubts about inflammation being a primary cause of laminitis, so it should be of no surprise to the reader when I advise caution in the use of NSAIDs for its treatment. I do recommend that they be used in the acute phase of laminitis, but suggest that the dose is reduced, and stopped, as soon as possible after this.

In acute laminitis, pain relief is imperative, and reducing the stress due to this will limit the effect on insulin sensitivity (*see* Chapter 8). Inflammation has been shown to occur in experimentally induced laminitis using BWE and with CHO (*see* Triggers, above).

This inflammatory response appears early in the developmental stage, and although pain seems only to occur once the laminae start to separate, inflammation may play a part in these cases. Beyond the acute stage, when the trigger has been removed or controlled, ongoing pain is much more likely to be the result of an unstable bone than due to inflammation. NSAIDs given at this stage can potentially result in more damage if the horse is made to feel comfortable and moves around too much on an unstable bone. This will be of particular concern if the horse's movement is not restricted, and even more so if hoof mechanics have not been addressed. In too many cases, the initial improvement seen as the laminae are repairing is followed by set-backs that are purely due to further mechanical damage rather than further episodes of active laminitis.

Another reason for reducing NSAID usage is the possibility of causing ulceration in the intestines. This would be unusual in normal horses on a maintenance dose, even with prolonged usage, but the risk increases significantly at higher doses.

Also sometimes used are salicylic acid (aspirin), Ketoprofen (Ketofen), Firocoxib (Equioxx), Maloxicam (Metacam), and in other countries, where it is available, intravenous DMSO is sometimes given for its reported anti-inflammatory properties. When the pain is particularly severe, the vet may have to try other medicines to control it.

Medication to Improve Blood Flow

Following the introduction of the theory that laminitis was caused by reduced blood perfusion through the capillaries, a range of drugs to try to cause vasodilation (to open blood vessels) and improve blood flow has been used. However, because vasodilation in the feet seems to be a feature of the developmental stage of laminitis, the use of any of these drugs appears to be contraindicated in the early stages of acute laminitis. Laminar blood vessels from laminitis cases have been shown to react abnormally to chemical stimulation, which could explain the lack of effectiveness of drugs given to try to achieve vasodilation.

ACP (Acetylpromazine, Acepromazine) is the most commonly used. ACP is a sedative, which can help to keep a horse calm to cope with the pain and the stress of being constantly stabled, but the reason it is given for laminitis is because it causes dilation of blood vessels (vasodilation). Although it appears that ACP produces vasodilation of the digital blood vessels, there is doubt that it actually increases laminar blood flow in laminitis.

Other medicines used include isoxsuprine, pentoxifylline, glyceryl trinitrate patches and Jiaogulan but none of these have been proven to be effective in the treatment of laminitis.

Other Medicines

There is insufficient space in this book to discuss the myriad of drugs, herbal remedies and supplements that have been, and still are being used as treatment for laminitis, a few of which may be of benefit to some horses, but many others probably of no use at all.

Because the damage occurs in the feet, we have been fooled into thinking that this is the area that needs to be treated, but I am optimistic that the change in direction – to find effective treatments for the triggers that cause laminitis, particularly insulin resistance – will give us a better chance of preventing laminitis from occurring.

MANAGEMENT OF LAMINITIS

In the acute phase, movement must be restricted, but it is difficult to know at what point, after this, the horse can be allowed more freedom to move. A number of considerations have to be made.

- Are the hoof capsule and sole adequately supported, and the hoof mechanics dealt with, to reduce the forces in the foot?
- There must be sufficient strength in the laminae to maintain the stability of P3 to withstand the increased forces of movement. Mild cases, where the laminae have just stretched and the basement membrane is mostly intact, can be allowed to walk within a couple of weeks. More severe cases, where there has been greater separation, will need significantly longer.
- In the sub-acute phase, pain is still a good indicator of instability of the bone, which may just be due to the severity of the initial attack, but could also show that the hoof mechanics have not been dealt with adequately.
- Before the horse is turned out, it should be off any pain-relieving medication. If the horse is not able to feel pain in the feet then it is liable to do more than it should, and thereby cause mechanical breakdown of the healing laminae. However, it may be safe to lead the horse out while on a low dose of 'bute', provided the hoof has been trimmed appropriately and the foot supported, and some people suggest that this might even be necessary for some IR horses, to increase the strength of the laminae and help the recovery process (*see* Chapter 8).
- If the palmar angle of P3 is high, either from trimming or from fitting wedges, the horse must remain confined until this angle has been reduced.
- In less severe cases, early on, horses may be very stiff when brought out of the box, but may then be seen to improve with walking. This is probably due to the foot movement pumping away oedema fluid that has collected. Oedema from increased fluid collection in the feet due to inflammation

has been suggested as the cause of laminitis, but there appears to be little evidence of this. The improvement seen as this fluid is removed from the laminae should not be misinterpreted, and the obvious decrease in lameness following this limited movement does not necessarily mean that more exercise will produce an even greater improvement, at this stage.

- Initially, controlled walking should be in straight lines and on a soft surface, which is more comfortable for the horse as well as being less likely to cause mechanical damage.

When the laminitic horse should be allowed greater movement is considered further under the management of insulin resistance in Chapter 8.

Stabling

Stabling the horse will be the most common means of confinement initially, and some consideration needs to be given to the bedding. If the horse is in a lot of pain, a deep bed should be provided so that it is able to lie down comfortably to take pressure off its sore feet, and so it is less likely to get bedsores. The choice of bedding used may depend on availability, cost, and whether external support is being provided on the feet, or other factors such as dust, or straw-eating leading to impaction, or sand being abrasive to the skin of horses that lie down a lot. If a horse is immobile, food and water need to be made accessible.

In the time between stabling and before pasture turnout, when the horse may have access to a restricted area, it is best if the surface is foot-conforming – for example soft ground, sand or pea-gravel – since this will reduce peripheral loading and lessen the breakover forces around the foot.

Diet

Diet is discussed in depth under the section concerning the management of insulin resistance in Chapter 8.

ATTENTION TO THE FEET

What should be done to the feet in the laminitis case is still an area where there are widely differing opinions. Foot treatment will often depend on an individual farrier's or vet's experience (of success and failure). It is likely to differ depending on the severity of the attack and the stage of the disease, and the cost of treatment might well also be a consideration.

Radiography can be of great benefit when dealing with laminitis, to assess damage, to help provide the correct trim (and shoe placement) and to monitor progress. Part of the reason that radiographs are not taken regularly will be financial, but there can be practical problems too, such as lack of power, the inability of the horse to stand, or to stand on a firm surface, or the availability of a level surface. Transporting a horse with acute laminitis is potentially very

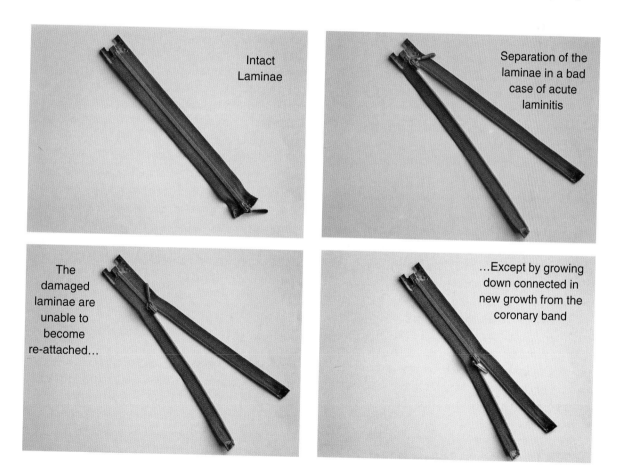

Intact Laminae

Separation of the laminae in a bad case of acute laminitis

The damaged laminae are unable to become re-attached…

…Except by growing down connected in new growth from the coronary band

Fig. 139 *The laminae of the dorsal hoof wall represented as a zip. In acute laminitis, the horny and sensitive laminae lose their connection and the two sides separate. Like a zip, the laminae are unable to reattach except by growing down together with new growth from the coronary band.*

damaging, and this must be a consideration if contemplating moving a laminitic horse – for example to a veterinary hospital – in order to have radiographs taken.

If the horse is shod, the shoes should probably be left on for a few days with the sole supported until the acute phase has passed, to try to avoid mechanical tearing of the laminae when attempting to remove the shoe, and in the opposite foot when more weight is transferred to it when doing so.

It is suggested that the feet of a horse suffering from acute laminitis should be put into ice (cryotherapy), but this only has been demonstrated to be of benefit in carbohydrate overload induced laminitis. (*See* Prevention of Laminitis, below.)

The trim is as important as what is subsequently applied to the foot. Most people suggest that the heels should be trimmed to lower the palmar angle of P3, to reduce the forces on to its tip, and to spread the load to the stronger, less damaged laminae at the heels. Also the toe should be shortened to make breakover easier, and to reduce the mechanical forces that tend to pull the hoof and bone apart when the horse moves.

Re-aligning the bone relative to the hoof, and reducing the forces acting on them both, allows laminae that have not completely separated to repair, and for the new hoof to grow down with laminae attached. These aims may be achieved by leaving the horse barefoot and managing it by trimming, sometimes with the use of boots and pads, because this allows the feet to be trimmed frequently without the trauma of re-shoeing. In other cases they may be accomplished with the application of shoes or hoof casts.

Do not forget about the hind feet: The effects of laminitis are seen most obviously in the front feet, and management generally concentrates on dealing with the problems in these feet. Because of this it is easy to forget that some changes will almost certainly have occurred in the hind feet as well.

Sole and Frog Support

Taped-on Styrofoam blocks or Stable Support System, pads in hoof boots, or EVA with Equicast may be used to support the sole and frog. Several options use 'impression' material to support the back half of the foot, which involves using two materials (of 'play-dough' consistency) that chemically react when mixed together, and set to produce a non-deformable but pliable form. This can be used with taped-on Stable Support System or Modified Ultimates, or with any shoe plus pad that is glued or nailed on, for example Epona Shoe, Steward Clog and EDSS.

If frog support is to be provided by fitting a metal heart-bar shoe, this should only be done following a radiograph for correct positioning, and to ensure that not too much pressure is put on to the frog. This is not so critical for the range of shoes in other materials that have a similar form because the 'tongue' portion is applied with neutral pressure and is not so rigid, for example Imprint Shoe, Epona Shoe.

Applying a plain shoe without providing any sole or frog support is likely to be detrimental in any case of laminitis.

Reducing the Forces of 'Breakover'

Although some devices applied to feet have rolled edges – for example, boots and Imprint Shoes – they extend beyond the perimeter of the foot so will be less effective at easing breakover. Some shoes will ease breakover just at the toe – for example Ultimates or 'reverse' shoes (shoes fitted with the branches towards the toe) – but others do so all around the foot, such as Steward Clog or EVA with Equicast, EDSS and Epona Shoe.

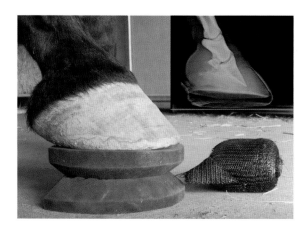

Fig. 140   An EVA + Equicast fulfil the requirements for dealing with the acute laminitis case; with the EVA providing sole support and reducing the forces of breakover and the Equicast providing stability to the hoof capsule. This method also has the advantage that the cast can be applied while the horse is standing on the EVA (by using a second EVA), thus minimizing the forces on the other foot, which can occur when other forms of support are applied. The EVA and cast can be seen on the radiograph of the foot of a horse with chronic laminitis. Compression of the front of the EVA is likely to be due to the way the foot was trimmed – the angle of the trim. (Radiograph courtesy Dave Richards)

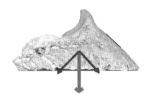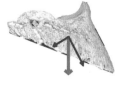

Fig. 141a   'Ground-parallel' bone with an even spread of load.

Fig. 142b   Twenty-degree palmar angle of P3, with loading of the tip of the bone.

Re-alignment of P3

Shoeing protocols that include a trimming method all appear to suggest trimming the heel to reduce the palmar angle of P3 – for example Imprint Shoes, Redden's Modified Ultimates and

EDSS; however, the last two of these then raise the heels with wedges or rails fitted to them, thus increasing the angle of the bone. Others raise the hoof angle but without suggesting a trim, such as the Outlaw boot, and sometimes fit on the Steward Clog.

The argument put forward for raising the hoof angle is to 'relieve the pull of the DDFT', which is blamed for the rotation of P3, and this is where there is disagreement with those who believe that the weight of the horse is of much more significance, of which I am one. A recent study using a biomechanical model system seems to agree with this, showing an increase in strain on the dorsal wall laminae as hoof angle is increased, and this is greatest in the proximal (top) wall. Trimming to lower the heels loads the back half of the foot and reduces the forces at the toe. The higher the bone angle, the more weight goes on to the tip of the bone, and the weight of the horse is constantly on it. The effect of the DDFT is likely to come into play when the horse moves, by pulling on the bone (away from the hoof) when the deep flexor muscle contracts. The effect of this can be reduced by easing breakover.

Stabilization of the Hoof Wall

If we try to open or separate something, we may well try to wiggle it to loosen attachments first. Having already lost some of its laminar connection, when the horse walks, extra movement of the hoof wall is likely to do a similar thing and cause more laminae to separate. Part of the benefit of using an Equicast, Imprint Shoe or Nolan Plate is likely to be by stabilizing the wall and helping to reduce this further laminar tearing. Shoes with nails will give the hoof some rigidity, but nail holes weaken the wall. One proposal involves grooving the hooves down the wall at the toe quarters. This may reduce the additional laminar tearing if the side walls are well connected, but would seem to be potentially catastrophic if they are not.

Being able to remove any appliance easily is of benefit by not causing damage to the wall, and allowing the hooves to be trimmed by a small amount more frequently, this being particularly important in chronic cases when the heels are growing faster than the toe.

MANAGING CHRONIC LAMINITIS

Far too many acute cases progress to chronic laminitis. Laminar repair, even in relatively mild cases, will leave the laminae weakened to some degree, and the overall strength of the laminae will be reduced after every further episode – but this is usually the result of, rather than the reason for, acute cases becoming chronic. There are four main reasons why so many acute cases become chronic.

● The trigger is large or not dealt with quickly enough, and laminar separation is extensive,

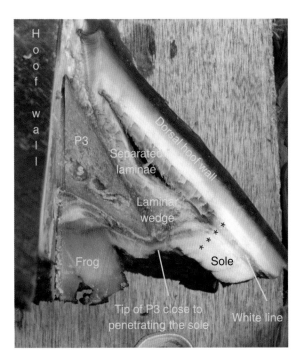

making recovery that much more difficult and taking longer for the laminae to 'recover'.

● The (over-)use of painkillers misleads owners, making them believe that their horse is getting better by allowing it to move more than the laminae are able to deal with. The horse may seem to be coping, but it only needs to have that 'silly moment' and things go badly wrong.

● IR is not dealt with, and the laminae continue to be weak and more prone to mechanical damage. IR not being controlled can be due to lack of knowledge, inability to deal with it, or insufficient commitment from the owner.

● Inappropriate trimming, or shoeing, that does not provide adequate support or sufficiently reduce the mechanical forces on the foot, makes the laminae more liable to damage when the horse moves.

Other physical changes also play a part. When a horse develops laminitis for the first time, the terminal papillae situated at the lower (distal) end of the laminae are distorted and new white line production is disrupted, but what was produced prior to the laminitis episode remains intact and attached to the sole and hoof wall (the 'ledge' in Fig. 142). When movement is restricted, this 'ledge' is able to support P3 sufficiently to allow the new hoof growth to stabilize the bone, and the horse seems to recover.

Healing can continue if the forces on the foot are kept under control, but as the hoof and ledge grow down and away from the bone, if the horse is allowed to do more than the repairing laminae can cope with, the tip of

Fig. 142 The hind foot of a horse six weeks after an acute laminitis attack. The tip of P3 has 'fallen off the ledge' (blue asterisks) and is about to penetrate the sole.

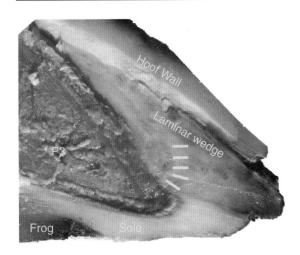

Fig. 143 *Chronic laminitic foot, with large laminar wedge. The short yellow lines (crescent) identify the terminal papillae that would normally produce the 'white line'. The tip of P3 is resting on the sole.*

the bone slips off the ledge to press directly on the sole, and the horse becomes severely lame again. It is not uncommon to hear of a horse which has had acute laminitis which has settled down, but having been let out on pasture, 'crashes' again at about six to eight weeks: this could well be due to this mechanical cause, rather than another active bout of laminitis.

Horses that have had laminitis often do not move so well on hard and uneven surfaces, and prefer to walk on the soft ground. This will be because P3 no longer has a ledge to support the tip of the bone, which therefore rests directly on the sole (Fig. 143.)

Further Complications of Laminitis

Laminitis 'Abscesses'

Laminitis 'abscesses' can occur following acute laminitis, but abscesses are also a problem in horses with chronic laminitis, when dirt and infection can gain entry to the foot through a

poorly formed 'white line'. These are dealt with in Chapter 11.

Sinker

The initial trigger may be so severe that it causes separation of the laminae all around the foot and the bone sinks inside the hoof capsule. It can also occur at a later stage, as a result of repeated laminitis episodes. Once support is lost from the dorsal wall, the forces acting on the rest of the foot will increase and can lead to separation further around the wall. When P3 sinks inside the hoof it takes the coronary band with it and causes the coronary papillae to bend, and this prevents new horn from growing down attached to the laminar corium (Fig. 144).

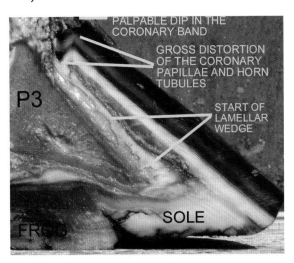

Fig. 144 *A 'sinker'. The bone sank six weeks prior to this photo, showing the coronary dip and gross distortion of the coronary papillae, as well as the start of laminar wedge.*

Sole Penetration

In some cases, the tip of P3 may penetrate the sole allowing infection to gain access to the damaged dermis, and to involve the bone as

Fig. 145 This cob was out on grass for five days after signs of lameness were first seen, by which time the bones had sunk in both front feet and the hind feet were also badly affected with laminitis. Certainly not a typical laminitic stance, 'standing under' on all four feet.

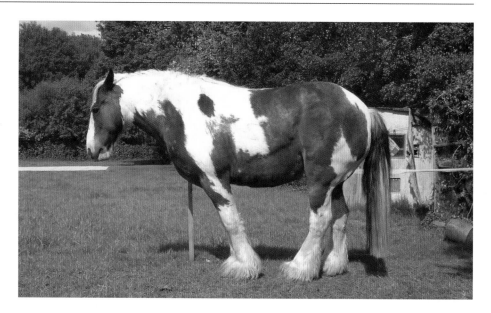

well. This occurs when the support in the front half of the foot has been lost and the weight of the horse is concentrated on the tip of the bone. The risk of penetration is increased significantly if there is pressure on the underside of the sole. When the sole is convex, it is very important not to allow it to make contact with the ground, or to receive any pressure from any impression material or pad applied to the sole

(*see* Fig. 146). Once penetration has occurred, some people use sterile maggots to help clean up the damaged and dead tissue.

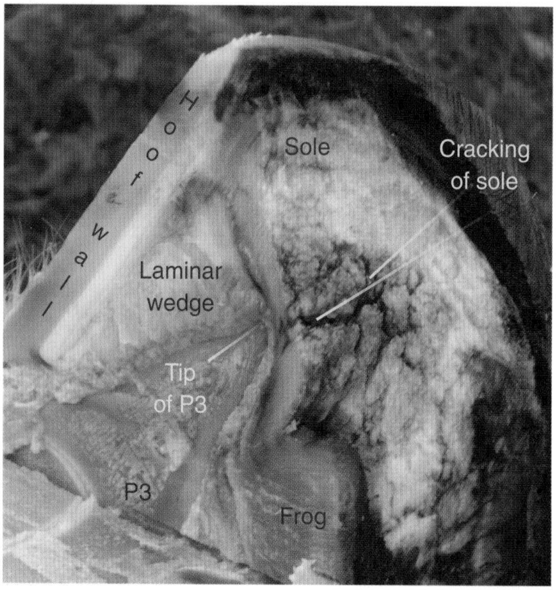

Uneven Medial and Lateral Separation

Another situation that can be extremely difficult to deal with is when there is uneven separation on the two sides of the foot and one side of the bone sinks down. This can occur if there is medio-lateral imbalance that unevenly loads the foot once the support from the dorsal wall is lost. The side wall (generally the medial wall) bends and is accompanied by narrower growth rings on that side.

Fig. 146 This horse developed laminitis in a hind foot following a severe injury to the other hind leg. The sole had become prominent and had started to crack underneath the tip of P3, which would shortly have penetrated the sole. The space between the hoof wall and P3 is filled by laminar wedge.

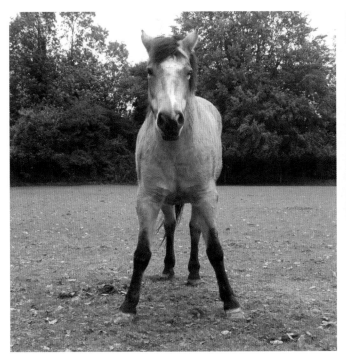

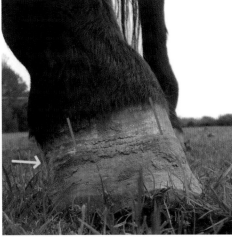

Fig. 147 *The left fore of the chronic laminitic pony in Fig. 127 during another 'acute episode'. The feet show slower growth on the medial side and a bend in the medial wall.*

Pain

Dealing with these complicated cases is made even more difficult by changes in the source of the pain, and in some chronic laminitis cases with constant pain it can be very difficult to work out what causes it. In some cases, the horse or pony responds to pain in the feet by tightening up the deep flexor muscle, in the same way that foals do to cause 'ballerina syndrome' (*see* Chapter 5), and this contracture can cause anoxia in the muscle, which itself is painful. Contracture of the muscle causes a constant tension in the DDFT, which prevents realignment of P3, and in these cases, trimming the heel leaves the horse standing on its toe with the heel unable to reach the ground. If de-rotation of P3 is not achieved by trimming and management, some vets will cut the inferior check ligament, or even the DDFT (*see* Deep Flexor Tenotomy below).

Another complication can be the development of neuropathic pain, which involves the sensitization of the pain receptors and intensifies the pain stimuli from the feet; however, it is hard to quantify the extent of this as a problem. This type of pain is very difficult to control.

Deep Flexor Tenotomy

DDFT tenotomy is a procedure that is advocated by several prominent vets, but one that I have no experience of. There are some reports of horses returning to work after this procedure, but it seems that, for the majority, 'pasture soundness' is the best that is achieved. Many of these horses will succumb to laminitis again because of the extensive laminar damage (that warranted the tenotomy to be done) and the problems of controlling IR, since they cannot be exercised. This has made it difficult for me to justify cutting such an important supporting structure of the leg. It does seem that many of those who regularly carry out these tenotomies are also the ones that treat acute laminitis by wedging up the feet, and I suspect that there is some connection, with one procedure eventually leading to the necessity of carrying out the other.

The Botox Option

Another option that is being tried, when de-rotation is not possible, is to inject very small doses of botulinum toxin (Botox) into the DDF muscle to paralyse it and stop the contracture, with the effect of this lasting about six months. The initial reports, from a few cases, was good and allowed de-rotation of P3, but the long-term success or failure will ultimately depend on the extent of damage in the feet and whether further damage can be prevented by correct management of these difficult cases.

The prognosis for many of these severely affected cases is not good and a successful outcome requires great skills from the vet and farrier and great commitment from an owner, requiring time, money and fortitude to survive the emotional roller-coaster.

PREVENTION OF LAMINITIS

For some time before I really started researching laminitis, I had suggested to owners that 'laminitis is rarely seen in horses and ponies that have regular exercise and regular foot trimming'. The reason for this can now be explained in that exercise helps to control IR, and regular hoof trimming limits the forces acting on the feet.

I suggest that the following precautionary measures should be taken in order to prevent laminitis.

● Preventing or controlling IR, by providing a suitable diet combined with exercise, will help to maintain stronger laminae (*see* Chapter 8).

● Do not let your horse become over-weight since this makes it more liable to developing IR and also increases the load on the feet.

● Limit grazing for IR horses, most importantly when the weather is very cold and sunny.

● If the horse has a long coat, or infections that are difficult to clear, test and/or treat for PPID.

● Ensure that the horse is not able to get into the feed-room.

● Keep the feet regularly trimmed, to limit the forces on the hoof wall and the laminae.

● Caution should be taken when considering the therapeutic administration of corticosteroids, particularly in IR horses (and PPID).

● Founderguard contains an antibiotic (virginiamycin) that is not absorbed from the intestines, and has been used to try to prevent the changes that occur in the large intestine as a result of high grain diets and of fructans in grass (Its availability is limited to certain countries).

● Support the sound foot if the opposite leg is badly injured and is too painful for the horse to use (This condition is more likely to be seen in a hospital situation).

● Check the source of wood-shavings to ensure they do not contain any from black walnut (This is not a problem in the UK).

● Cryotherapy (ice treatment) has been shown to limit the extent of laminar changes following oligofructose overdose. It does not completely stop any changes, but limits them sufficiently to prevent clinical laminitis.

Cryotherapy

It seems that cryotherapy is increasingly being advocated as a 'first aid measure' in the treatment of laminitis, but I have doubts about how efficacious this is likely to be in many cases of laminitis, for both physiological and practical reasons. For laminitis caused by CHO (carbohydrate-induced laminitis), it is thought that cryotherapy 'prevents' it by limiting access of the laminitis trigger by reducing blood flow, and by decreasing the activity of the MMP enzymes; also cryotherapy has now been shown to be of benefit once clinical laminitis has started in CHO-induced laminitis (*see* Chapter 12). However, laminitis may be a result of venoconstriction in IR-induced laminitis, so cryotherapy could potentially worsen the situation. (Some people report that their IR/laminitis horses are more sore in freezing temperatures in winter.)

Other suggested benefits of cryotherapy are that the cold temperatures reduce inflammation and pain; however, inflammation does not appear to be a significant feature in IR-induced laminitis.

There are serious practical difficulties in employing the methods used experimentally, which is keeping the horse's legs in large ice-boots or in an ice-bath for several days. Questions to ask are whether other methods achieve sufficiently cold temperatures to have any effect, and could intermittent cooling actually be detrimental? Experimentally, temperature reduction of the feet was found to be more effective when ice and water reached midway up the cannon than if below the fetlock. It seems unlikely that intermittently putting the feet in bags of ice will reduce the foot temperature sufficiently.

8 Insulin Resistance (IR) and Low Grade Laminitis

Insulin resistance (IR) describes an altered metabolic state that occurs in many mammals, particularly if they are overweight, and is of particular importance in man because it can progress to Type 2 diabetes, and in horses because of its involvement in laminitis. IR occurs most commonly in obese individuals in man, horses and other species; however, it is not restricted only to those who are overweight, and not all obese individuals are insulin resistant.

Adipocytes (fat cells) are not just stores of fat in the body: they also release hormones and other substances into the blood, and certain types of fat are recognized as being more hormonally active – for example, abdominal fat in man. We can recognize IR in horses from the clinical sign of abnormal fat deposits over the body, particularly involving the neck ('cresty neck'), and there is some evidence that fat at this site differs in activity from other sites.

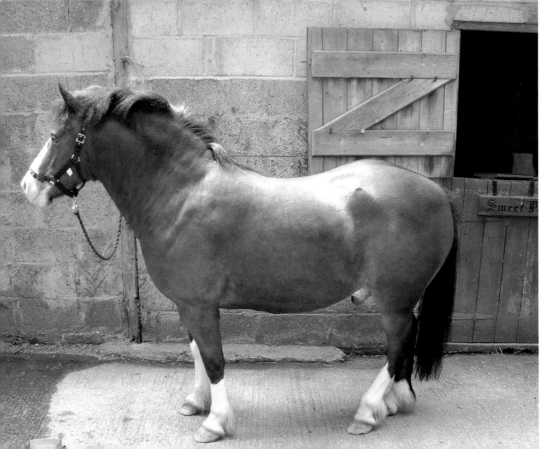

Fig. 148 An obese, insulin-resistant pony.

Certain races of people and certain breeds of horse are more prone to developing IR. For horses, the explanation is put forward that they evolved to live in tough environments, and that the metabolic changes of IR allowed them to put on weight when food was plentiful to provide the reserves required for when food was scarce. Man has completely changed the situation for these horses and ponies, providing energy-rich food throughout the year and removing the necessity for them to travel distances (and exercise themselves) to search for it. IR can be considered a normal metabolic process for these 'native breeds', but the management systems to which we subject them do not allow them to control it.

In a similar way, lack of exercise and a modern diet of energy-rich food (and alcohol) have resulted in the explosion in the numbers of obese, insulin-resistant humans.

WHAT IS INSULIN RESISTANCE?

Decreased insulin sensitivity = increased insulin resistance

Insulin is produced by the pancreas, and its production and release is increased after eating, mainly in response to the absorption of sugars from the small intestine. It is necessary for the body to maintain constant levels of glucose in the blood, and insulin helps to control this by facilitating glucose uptake by cells and helping tissues to store any excess as glycogen.

Glucose is used by cells to provide energy, but it cannot just pass from the blood directly through the cell wall: it has to go through a 'gate'. Different cells have different types of gate, but the ones of interest in IR are those that require insulin to open them (GLUT4). In IR, the opening mechanism becomes less sensitive, and more insulin is required to open these gates, and significantly greater amounts are produced to enable glucose uptake by these cells. The

cells of many tissues have glucose transport systems that are not dependant on insulin, but important ones that do are muscle, fat and liver cells.

THE PANCREAS

The pancreas is a glandular organ that produces digestive enzymes and hormones that help the body to chemically break down, digest and utilize food. It lies very close to the top of the small intestine (the duodenum), and the pancreatic duct opens into it. Insulin and glucagon are two of the hormones produced by the pancreas that are particularly involved in controlling blood glucose levels.

In Type 1 diabetes in people, insulin production by the pancreas is impaired, so that the cells requiring insulin for glucose uptake are unable to do so, and this causes the blood glucose level to rise and remain dangerously high. Those that suffer from this form of diabetes must provide their body with the necessary insulin to deal with this, and do so with daily injections.

Significantly, those suffering from Type 1 diabetes are aware that exercise increases glucose uptake by muscle cells, independent of insulin, so in order to prevent post-exercise hypoglycaemia (dangerously low blood glucose), they must either reduce the dose of insulin they inject, or increase their food intake.

In Type 2 diabetes in people the pancreas, which prior to this was able to produce sufficient insulin to maintain normal glucose levels, becomes unable to keep up with the constant demand for high levels of insulin in IR, which leads to the pancreas becoming 'exhausted'. Insulin injections will be needed if the IR is not controlled and insulin production in the pancreas fails.

Many human patients do not progress to Type 2 diabetes because they are able to change their life-style to reduce the demands on the pancreas. In simple terms, they do so by changing to a low-sugar diet and by increasing exercise. Smaller amounts of sugar in the diet require less insulin to be produced to maintain constant blood glucose levels, and exercise improves glucose uptake by cells, reducing the requirement for insulin to do so.

In the insulin-resistant horse, the pancreas, in most cases, is able to maintain the higher production of insulin that is required, thus avoiding Type 2 diabetes, but the very high levels of insulin appear to cause changes in the laminae.

The way that overweight horses are still commonly managed – changing their diet mostly by restriction, and confining them to stables or small areas – in no way addresses the underlying IR problem. We need to correctly address the dietary needs of these horses, with particular attention to providing them with a 'low sugar' diet and, wherever possible, to increase their exercise.

THE CLINICAL SYMPTOMS OF IR

The clinical (physical) symptoms of IR include the following.

- A prominent and firm crest on the neck: this is the most obvious symptom associated with IR. A hard and immovable neck crest indicates that IR is not under control, and should set off alarm bells that something urgently needs to be done to control it. A neck crest that is soft and movable is a reasonable indicator that insulin resistance is relatively under control, but while there is still an obvious crest, IR control measures must be maintained.

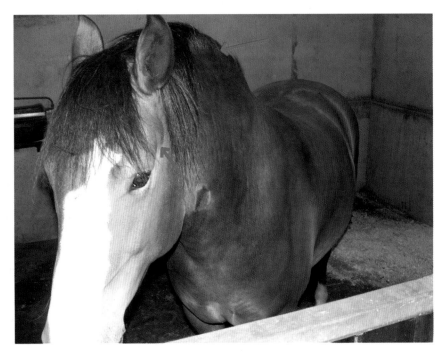

Fig. 149 A fat, insulin-resistant Welsh pony with a large neck crest and bulging of the supra-orbital fossa.

- Abnormal deposits of fat elsewhere on the body – for example over the tail-head and in front of mammary glands or prepuce, over the loins and behind the shoulders – are common and obvious signs of IR
- Fat deposits in the supra-orbital fossa, causing a bulge above the eyes (where normally there is a hollow)
- Laminitis is common in IR horses and ponies
- Changes are sometimes evident in the feet without apparently having caused lameness, such as obvious growth rings on the hooves, or a widened 'white line' (*see* Chapter 9, IR Rings and White Line Disease). The term 'low grade laminitis' is sometimes used to refer to these changes.
- An increase in appetite
- Infertility

Sometimes we are presented with a horse or pony with laminitis that the owner insists has never had it before, but the changes in the feet tell a different story. There may be obvious growth rings, deviation of the dorsal wall or widening of the white line, all evidence that the horse has had a low grade laminitis for some time. It may be that the owner has not noticed that the horse was lame, but intermittent, low grade weakening of the laminae seems to be able to produce these changes without the horse or pony showing obvious lameness.

Laminitis can be caused experimentally by giving large amounts of insulin, through an intravenous drip, to horses and ponies, and it appears to occur as a direct result of the high blood insulin levels. Although the insulin levels in these experiments is significantly higher than is found in the vast majority of IR cases we see,

further experiments have shown changes in the laminae at insulin levels that are often found in IR horses and ponies.

Increased levels of insulin, whether from an intravenous drip or from the fluctuations in production in the IR horse in response to a diet high in simple sugars and starch, cause weakening of the laminae, sufficient to produce clinical laminitis in some cases, or low grade laminitis when less damage occurs.

The Changes Occurring in the Feet

In man, the peripheral effects of IR cause changes in the blood circulation, and it would appear that this is also the case in horses. The action of insulin on blood vessels is normally to cause vasodilation, but in IR it produces the opposite effect, and vasoconstriction occurs.

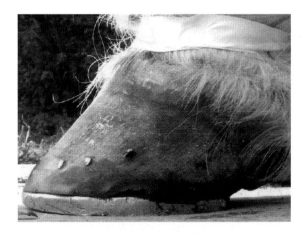

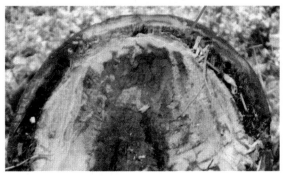

Fig. 150 Acute laminitis in a Welsh Section D pony, which reputedly had never had laminitis before. The changes in the hoof are not so easy to see, but there is obvious widening of the 'white line' and splits in it (arrow), which is evidence that the pony had low grade laminitis prior to the acute laminitis.

The effect of the reduction in blood flow on the laminae appears to be due to glucose deprivation rather than ischaemia (oxygen deprivation).

In insulin-induced laminitis, it is the integrity of the basal cell layer attached to the basement membrane that is affected.

IR causes weakening of the laminae, in that when a horse becomes insulin resistant the areas of attachment between basal cells are reduced, and the laminae become weaker (*see* Chapter 12); however, if IR is controlled the damage is repaired and the laminae become stronger again. Healthy feet can normally withstand any forces they are subjected to, but if the laminae are weakened, they will be less capable of doing so. The consequence of this will depend on the extent of the laminar weakening, and the forces they are subjected to.

When a horse has had laminitis previously, almost inevitably the 'repaired' laminae will be weaker than normal, and will become progressively weaker after every bout of laminitis. Furthermore, the greater the mechanical forces acting on the feet, the more likely it is that the weakened laminae will separate. The following factors will affect these mechanical forces.

● The fatter the horse, the more weight the feet have to cope with.
● The faster a horse moves, the greater the forces on the laminae.
● The harder the ground, the greater the peripheral loading on the hoof wall and the laminae.
● Longer periods of exercise increase the forces on the feet.
● The way the feet are trimmed will affect laminar loading.
● How frequently the feet are trimmed will also affect the forces acting on the feet.

THE METABOLIC CHANGES THAT CAUSE IR

Although IR has been recognized as a metabolic disease for some time, it is only relatively recently that its significance, in both man and horse, has been realized. How IR develops, and how it produces its effects, have not yet been identified, but there are some findings that appear to explain what we see in this form of laminitis.

The three things that appear to be the favourites to cause IR to develop are adipokines, cortisol, and insulin itself, and their effects are all interrelated. Adipokines refer to hormones and other proteins produced and released from certain types of fat.

Adipokines

The metabolic changes brought about by adipokines are complex and not fully understood, but with greater fat deposits there is increased production of leptin, resistin, pro-inflammatory cytokines and a reduction in the appetite-controlling hormone adiponectin, all of which have been implicated in contributing to insulin resistance. (Although leptin output is increased, its 'appetite-reducing' effect seems to be limited in IR because there can also be an associated reduced leptin sensitivity, referred to as leptin resistance.)

The relevance of this is that the fatter the horse, the more adipokines will be produced. The effects of leptin and adiponectin on controlling hunger are reduced, accounting for the increased appetite in insulin-resistant horses and ponies.

Cortisol and Insulin

Fat tissue produces an enzyme that is able to convert the 'inactive' corticosteroid cortisone

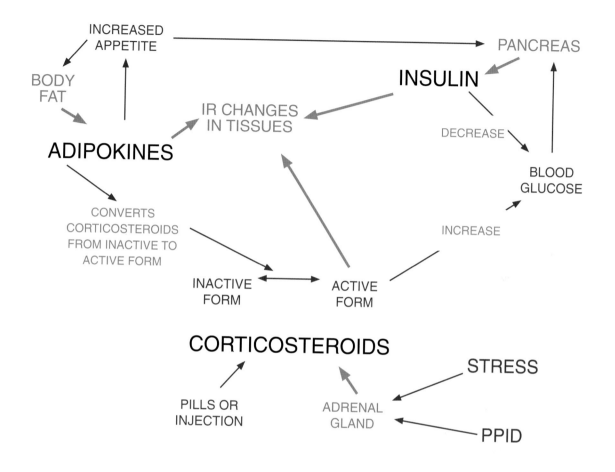

Fig. 151   The possible involvement of adipokines, insulin and corticosteroids in insulin resistance.

into the 'active' cortisol, thus increasing the effects of corticosteroids. Corticosteroids counteract the effects of insulin in two ways: they alter the metabolism of carbohydrates, fats and proteins, as well as having a direct effect on cells to reduce the sensitivity of the insulin receptors. Corticosteroids cause blood glucose to rise, which stimulates an increase in insulin production.

The relevance of this is that conditions that increase levels of corticosteroids in the body will have an effect on IR. PPID (*see* later), stress or corticosteroids given for treatment can cause IR, or worsen any existing IR.

High levels of insulin appear to cause decreased sensitivity of the glucose transport system GLUT4 in the tissues, and cause insulin resistance.

ASSESSING BODY CONDITION

A means of assessing the fatness of a horse would seem to be necessary, since surveys have identified that a large number of owners are unaware that their fat horses are overweight. Fat horses are more likely to develop foot changes due to the

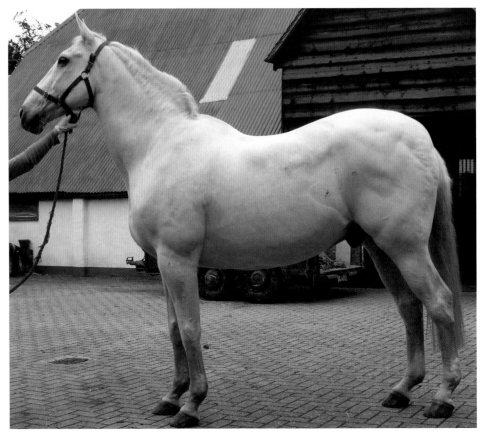

Fig. 152 Insulin-resistant horses may have a less obvious cresty neck than pony breeds, but they still have abnormal deposits of fat. Condition score 4/5.

higher amounts of adipokines produced, contributing to IR, and their extra bodyweight causing greater loading of the laminae.

Although a weigh-tape is useful to monitor a horse's weight gain or loss, it does not necessarily indicate whether it is overweight, since this depends on the size of the horse or pony.

Body Condition Scoring

Estimation of the fat cover on the neck, over the back, ribs and rump by manual palpation can be used to give a 'score' when compared to defined parameters, with a lower figure being given to thin horses and a higher one if it is fat. Different

scoring systems have been devised: 0 to 5, 1 to 5, or 1 to 9, with the median figure being described as 'moderate' or 'good condition'. My preference would be to use 1 to 5, with a score of 3 having:

- No crest on the neck
- The ribs just covered but easily felt
- The backbone well covered, but the spinous processes easily felt
- The rump rounded, but the pelvis easily felt

Using a body score grading of 1 to 5 would seem to simplify the risk assessment for IR, where 1 is emaciated, 2 is underweight, 3 means 'in good condition', 4 is overweight and at greater risk of IR, and 5 is obese and at extreme risk of IR.

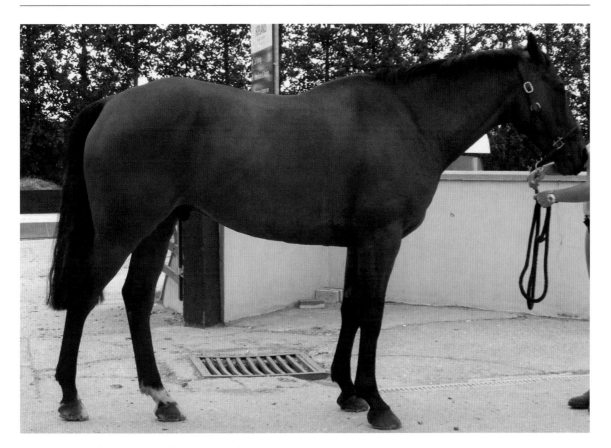

Fig. 153 Condition score 3 (in 1 to 5 scoring).

Unfortunately 'good condition' is too commonly used to refer to horses with a score of 4. It can only be hoped that show judges will eventually realize that by rewarding fat horses in the ring they are encouraging owners to put their horses at risk.

CARBOHYDRATES IN THE DIET

It is not just the *amount* of carbohydrate ingested by the horse, but also the type of carbohydrate that needs to be controlled in IR horses. Plant carbohydrates include cellulose, hemicelluloses and pectins, which form the outer structure of the plant, (structural carbohydrates, or SCs) and those that are used by the plant, or stored for use when they are needed (non-structural carbohydrates, or NSCs).

Structural carbohydrates steadily increase as the plant grows, whereas the NSC content of grass is extremely variable, depending to a great extent on environmental conditions. There are two forms of storage sugars in plants, with most plants storing extra sugar as starch (chains of glucose units), but others, including the grasses in the UK, storing the extra sugar as fructan (chains of fructose units).

The selection of grasses for pastures has

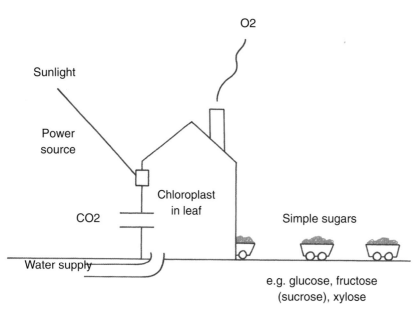

Fig. 154   The energy from the sun converts carbon dioxide and water into simple sugars and oxygen in the leaves of plants.

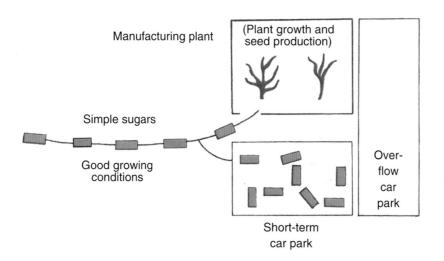

Fig. 155   When it is warm and sunny, the plant produces large quantities of simple sugar, which it uses to grow and for seed production. In warm conditions, the 'car park' empties overnight.

generally been aimed at putting weight on cattle (and sheep), choosing types that are efficient at producing carbohydrates that enable the grass to grow rapidly. Much of the cultivated pasture in the UK has been planted with grass species (particularly ryegrass) that are very efficient at forming simple sugars, and storing any excess as fructan in adverse climatic conditions. The grasses in pasture in hotter climates ('warm-season' grasses), clover and forage legumes (alfalfa) store excess sugars as starch. Even in plants that store sugars as fructan, the sugar stored in seeds is starch.

Fig. 156 If growth is slowed or stops (in the UK this is generally due to low temperatures), although fewer sugars are produced, they are in excess of requirements and are stored by the plant.

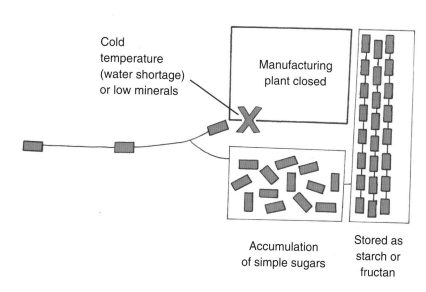

Cold temperature (water shortage) or low minerals

Manufacturing plant closed

Accumulation of simple sugars

Stored as starch or fructan

Carbohydrate Digestion in the Horse

The horse evolved to rely on the microbial digestion of the structural carbohydrates in plants for much of its energy requirements, rather than NSCs, which are extremely variable and would generally make up only a limited part of their diet. However, the horse is able to make use of these NSCs, when plentiful, by altering its metabolism and becoming insulin resistant, so that it can convert them to glycogen and fat as energy stores in the body for times when food is scarce.

The horse does not have enzymes in its intestines that can break down the structural carbohydrates of plants, and relies on the microbial population in its caecum and large intestine (hindgut) to ferment these carbohydrates, breaking them down to form volatile fatty acids (weak acids). For the storage sugars, virtually all of the fructan and variable amounts of starch are also fermented

in the hindgut, producing lactic acid (a stronger acid).

The amount of starch broken down into its glucose units, and absorbed from the small intestine, depends on several factors: the type of starch, the amount of starch, the timing of intake (of grain, in relation to forage), how it is processed (for grain), and individual differences between horses. The glucose from starch breakdown, and the other simple sugars, are absorbed through the small intestine and stimulate the release of insulin from the pancreas.

'Pasture-related' Laminitis

A large percentage of laminitis cases, particularly in the UK, are 'pasture related'. Currently there are two explanations why horses on grass pasture develop laminitis: the first is that high levels of fructan from grass pass

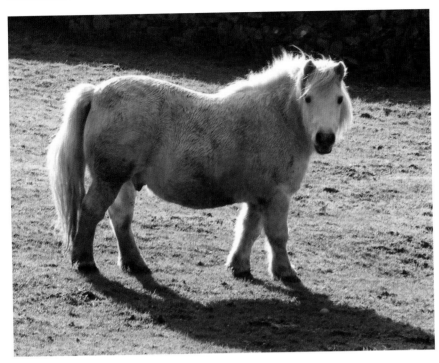

Fig. 157 An insulin-resistant pony with 'low grade laminitis'; this wasn't noticed because he was never exercised and just stood around in the field, eating.

through the small intestine into the hindgut, where they produce changes in the gut flora and cause the pH to fall sufficiently to cause the gut wall to be damaged. This allows the escape of a trigger factor (or factors) that activates MMP enzymes in the feet, to cause laminar separation and clinical laminitis.

The second is that high levels of simple sugars (and seed starch) in grass are absorbed through the small intestine, causing insulin to be released from the pancreas. The high levels of simple sugars in grass (as a result of heavy pasture growth, or when environmental conditions limit growth) produce a greater insulin response, to cause, or worsen, IR. This results in low-grade laminitis in some horses, and clinical laminitis in others.

There seems to be a move towards the 'metabolic/IR theory' and away from the MMP-activation theory, because although this is generally accepted as the reason laminitis occurs after a horse gets into the feed-room, and when laminitis is produced experimentally with oligofructose overdose, there are some who doubt that horses can ingest sufficient fructan from pasture to develop laminitis. In situations when there are very high levels of fructan in grass, there are also higher amounts of simple sugars, and although I personally believe that both of these mechanisms are able to cause laminitis in horses and ponies on pasture in some circumstances, it is more likely that they do so in conjunction with each other. (This is discussed further in Chapter 12.)

The Influence of Exercise

Horses on cultivated pasture need to do less walking for a greater intake of grass, making them more likely to put on weight and become insulin resistant. In my experience, the difference between those fat horses and ponies out at pasture that develop laminitis, and those that don't, is exercise. Those that are exercised regularly are generally saved from laminitis, and those that don't have exercise are the ones that succumb to it. Glucose uptake in muscle is increased by exercise, reducing the need for the pancreas to produce such high levels of insulin.

Why I feel that all fat horses need to have a change in their management is that those that have regular exercise have their IR under control (sometimes referred to as 'compensated IR'), but it only needs a change in circumstances, when the horse is unable to be exercised for a period of time, for IR to become 'uncompensated' and for laminitis to occur. It may be when the owner goes on holiday for two weeks and the horse is not ridden, or the horse goes lame for some other reason, so cannot be exercised but is still turned out to pasture, which tips the balance.

If IR causes weakening of the laminae by breaking down basal cell bonds (*see* Chapter 12), it will not be a static process, and the bonds will reconstruct when IR is controlled, and break down when it is not controlled. Those horses that have regular exercise are more likely to have their IR under control and have stronger laminae. The weaker laminae in the feet of those that are not exercised may be able to cope with the relatively small forces on them from just walking around, and it may actually be exercise in these horses that sets off clinical laminitis. This is because the weakened laminae may be unable to cope with the additional forces, or it may be the extra mechanical forces on feet that have been left too long that causes laminar breakdown.

Thus after their two weeks holiday, the owner should not take their fat horse out for a vigorous three-hour ride, because the laminae may have been weakened too much to cope with this. Overweight horses need to be brought back into work slowly to allow the basal cell bonds to regenerate and strengthen, to enable the laminae to cope with the increased forces. The feet need to be trimmed regularly to reduce the forces acting on the laminae, and if overgrown, should be attended to before the exercise

regime of a fat horse is significantly increased. Some cases of 'road founder' will be in IR horses, whose feet are not able to cope with the forces on them because of weakened laminae.

DIAGNOSIS OF IR

A diagnosis of IR can be made if a horse or pony is overweight or obese and has a cresty neck and regional adiposity. In other circumstances, a horse may need to be blood tested to confirm IR, to estimate the degree of IR, or to differentiate it from PPID, which can share the symptoms (*see* later in this chapter).

There are some problems diagnosing IR through blood testing, with the most efficient tests being generally impractical other than in hospital and laboratory situations and the 'field tests' available being somewhat unreliable, and the interpretation of them by vets, one has to say, rather inconsistent.

In insulin-resistant horses, the release of insulin from the pancreas following feeding is greater and lasts longer than in normal horses, so that if a raised serum insulin level is found in a blood test from a horse that has been starved overnight, it is highly suggestive of IR. Taking a blood sample to test for this is simple and relatively inexpensive, but not specific or very sensitive since a number of factors can affect insulin levels – not least how recently the horse has eaten, but also in response to pain, illness and stress (for instance when a horse is suffering from laminitis).

Due to variations in NSC, and thus the insulin response, it is far more difficult to interpret blood results from horses that have been out on pasture or given untested hay prior to the blood test, so 'fasting overnight' is generally recommended before blood testing. This has the advantage of being easily repeatable for comparison with follow-up tests, but may produce higher than normal figures if a horse, normally at pasture, is stressed by being stabled, and IR horses that have a low basal insulin level but have an exaggerated response to food, may be missed.

Some people use the blood glucose to insulin ratio to diagnose IR, which does appear to improve the reliability of the results. Some vets try to improve the consistency of the test by assessing a horse's response to a dose of dextrose (glucose), which involves this being given with some chaff by the owner, with the vet attending two hours later to collect the blood sample.

High levels of triglycerides may be found in the blood in IR, particularly in ponies, with triglyceride testing being part of the protocol for IR diagnosis in man.

PREVENTION AND MANAGEMENT OF IR

The prevention of IR relies on weight management of the horse, providing a diet low in NSCs, and ensuring the horse has regular exercise. In many cases, owners only discover their horse is insulin resistant once it has developed laminitis, and in these cases, management of IR has to rely on strict dietary management since control of IR by exercise, certainly initially, is no longer an option.

Weight Management

The condition score of horses should be monitored, and the availability of food should be altered accordingly.

The availability of convenient feeds and the marketing power of feed manufacturers has resulted in many horses receiving inappropriate diets that contribute to their obesity and IR. A forage diet is adequate for the requirements of very many horses and ponies. Horses that have greater energy requirements may not be able to obtain enough energy from just forage,

because it is not sufficiently energy dense and there is a limit to how much grass or hay can be eaten. For these horses, additional 'hard feed' should be tailored to their needs, and should be reduced if exercise is reduced due to injury or adverse weather conditions.

Overweight horses need to have their food intake controlled to enable them to lose weight, but one of the clinical effects of IR is an increased appetite, which makes control of a horse's weight more difficult, particularly when they are out at pasture or when given ad lib hay. For those out on pasture, grass intake can be reduced by giving them less time on pasture, or turning them out on a 'dirt patch'. Neither of these is particularly satisfactory for a horse that is insulin resistant, because they limit the horse's movement. If a horse accepts having a grazing muzzle on, it can still be turned out with its companions and will generally move around more while trying to find grass that it can eat through the muzzle.

Insulin-resistant horses that have already developed laminitis will initially be confined to a stable, and it will be necessary to limit their hay in order for them to lose weight.

In the past, horses with laminitis were removed from pasture and their food severely restricted, but this should be avoided, particularly in overweight ponies and donkeys, since the consequences can be life-threatening due to hyperlipidaemia (meaning 'too much – fat – in the blood'), which can affect their liver and other organs. This occurs due to the breakdown of fats to provide energy, if they obtain insufficient energy from their diet. For an obese horse, the suggested amount of low sugar hay it should be given is either 1.5 per cent of the horse's current weight, or 2 per cent of what its 'ideal' bodyweight should be, whichever is the greater. The horse's neck crest, fat deposits and body condition score should all be monitored, and the quantity of hay given should be adjusted according to the response to the restriction in diet.

For a horse that consumes its hay rapidly, there can be metabolic as well as practical benefits in providing the hay in some form of 'slow feeder', with the use of small-mesh bags or haynets such as a 'Hay Pillow' in order to reduce the rate of consumption.

Restriction of Carbohydrate Intake

IR horses need to have their access to pasture controlled, not just because of the amount of grass, but also because of the variability of the NSC content. There are some circumstances when NSC levels may be 'safe' and other situations when no access should be allowed (*see* box 'Pasture NSCs' later in this chapter).

CARBOHYDRATE TESTING

Abbreviations used when testing for carbohydrates:

ESC (Ethanol-soluble carbohydrates) = simple sugars + short-chained fructans

WSC (Water-soluble carbohydrates) = ESC + long-chained fructans

NSC = WSC + Starch

For laminitis cases, pasture will not be an option and the horse should be provided with a high-fibre, 'low-sugar' diet, which is generally hay but may be haylage and can include alfalfa or unmollassed sugar beet. Although hay will have lower NSC levels than the grass it was cut from, if these were high at the time, these products may still have NSC levels that are dangerous for the IR horse. Where practical, hay should be tested: an NSC below 10 per cent is considered safe for IR horses. Taking core

samples from a number of bales will give an indication of the sugar content, and can also provide information about minerals, vitamins, protein and so on. Different labs will test for different sugar groups, and it is important to understand what results they are reporting. Some labs will only provide results for ESC plus starch, but this is probably not suitable for our situation in the UK, and although some hays may have WSC and ESC that are very similar, sometimes the difference between the two (which is the long-chained fructans) can be significant.

Freshly produced haylage can be high in NSCs so should be avoided, but will usually be safe once it has 'cured', after fermentation has used up some of its sugar. Alfalfa harvested in other countries can have higher starch and sugar levels than are found in the UK, which might account for reports of horses having relapses when given it, but also could be due to an individual's response to it; either way some care should be taken when this is used as part of the diet. In the UK it is generally given to horses incorporated in proprietary feeds.

If it is not possible or practical to test the hay, the levels of water-soluble carbohydrate (simple sugars and fructans, but not starch) can be reduced by soaking; reported to be as much as 30 per cent if soaked in hot water for half an hour, or rather longer in cold water. Soaking the hay for longer is unlikely to reduce the sugars much more, and may affect the quality of the hay and its palatability. Of course, make sure that the horse has no access to the discarded 'sugar water'.

Grain should be avoided as well as high NSC proprietary feeds and anything with added molasses, and if you 'must' give tit-bits, then ones with low sugar should be used. Apples and carrots are unnecessary and should be avoided.

Unmollassed sugar beet can be used to replace some of the hay, and in the UK we are lucky to have a number of feed companies committed to producing forage and mixes low

PASTURE NSCS

NSCs in plants vary from day to day and hour to hour. NSCs will be **higher (in bold)** in some situations than others (*lower in italics*) – though note that although these *'lower'* levels are safer than the situations when they might be **'higher'**, they can still be unsafe for an IR horse!

● Improved (cultivated) pasture will have higher NSCs than *rough pasture* under the same climatic conditions, due to the type of grasses in it.

Sunlight enables the plant to manufacture sugars, therefore:

● NSCs are *not produced at night.*
● NSCs will be *lower when it is cloudy*, and when it is sunny, *in shaded areas of pasture* even in long grass (which shades itself).
● More NSCs are produced when the daylight is longer (but usage will generally also be greater).
● When it is sunny, NSCs will tend to build up over the day, so will be **higher in the late afternoon** than *first thing in the morning* (from plant usage overnight ** *see* below).
● **'Bald patches' that are green get full sunshine and may be 'stressed', so can have high NSCs.**
● To be effective (and safe), *'bald patches' need to be mostly dirt.*

Temperature will affect the balance of NSC manufacture and usage:

● NSCs *are generally lower in warmer weather* in the grass types in the UK.
● **In cold sunny weather, NSCs can increase to dangerous levels, particularly for the IR horse (** for each consecutive cold sunny day, NSCs will be higher each morning)**
● NSCs in warm-season grasses (not the UK) and alfalfa are generally higher in hot conditions (when water or minerals are limited).
● *Fertilized pasture is likely to be lower in NSC* than unfertilized pasture (improves usage over manufacture), **but there is likely to be a lot more grass.**
● **Lack of water can stress the plant.** The effect of long-term drought can cause rises in NSC, depending on the species and variety of grass, and the duration of the drought.
● **When the seed is being formed,** horses may **selectively graze** the top of the plant (where the seed is).
● Some weeds may be high in NSCs, for example the dandelion.
● **Pasture immediately after hay cutting could be very high in NSCs** (since these are stored in the stems), until the NSCs have been used up in new leaf growth. A similar situation may occur with over-grazed pasture.

ALL PLANTS, IN CERTAIN CONDITIONS, CAN HAVE AMOUNTS OF NSC DANGEROUS FOR IR HORSES

in NSC (look for the 'Laminitis Trust Approval Mark for horse feeds').

Some feeds are advertised as suitable for laminitis cases but actually contain more than 10 per cent NSC, which actually also applies to some feeds with the Laminitis Trust Mark. Although the Laminitis Trust has strict guidelines that feed manufacturers must follow to obtain the 'Trust Mark', which includes limits on NSC, because the guidelines refer to NSC levels 'when fed at the recommended rate', some products with the mark have NSC over 10, so need to be used with caution. If it does not tell you the NSC levels on the bag it is advisable to phone the manufacturer to find out the NSC content, and if they cannot tell you, then do not feed it.

Supplementation of minerals and vitamins is recommended, particularly in these cases when the diet is restricted. This is aimed at maintaining the overall health of the horse and not just IR. Without hay testing, we have little idea of what supplementation is required, and manufactured supplements may have to be relied upon. A number of minerals have been suggested to be of benefit in IR in humans – for example supplementing magnesium and chromium in the diet – but there is no more than anecdotal evidence of their benefit in horses. Magnesium is often low in the spring and autumn when the grass is growing rapidly, and these are times that we commonly see laminitis, so supplementation of this, particularly at these times of year, could well be of benefit.

By taking a horse off pasture, we may be depriving it of the benefits of its natural forage, but it does allow greater control over what it eats. It gives the opportunity to provide a fixed amount of food of known quality, and the ability to provide and balance the vitamins and minerals it is getting, but this does need a fair amount of commitment on the part of the owner. Some horses that develop laminitis and can have no exercise, may need this level of dietary control.

Exercise

The amount of exercise required to keep IR under control will depend on the breed of horse or pony and how well the diet is managed. For most horses and ponies, 'regular exercise' should be, at a minimum, exercise every other day. This does not necessarily need to be hard work and can just be brisk walking, provided it is sufficient to increase the circulation in the feet.

For IR horses that have developed laminitis and still have an unstable P3, exercise cannot be used to control IR because movement will cause further laminar separation, so at this stage horses must be restricted, and management of IR has to rely on very strict control of the diet.

Because very many cases of laminitis have IR as an underlying problem, keeping these horses confined for weeks may not be the best way to deal with them unless IR is fully controlled by diet. If IR isn't controlled, the basal cell layer will remain unstable and the laminar attachment of the new growth, and of those that have repaired, will remain weaker, leaving the horse more prone to relapse when it is eventually allowed out.

Movement has beneficial effects on the healing process in those laminitic feet that are able to withstand the increased forces, by improving circulation and helping to control IR, *but only if they are able to withstand the increased forces.*

The Reintroduction of Exercise

As stability returns and the pain subsides, controlled walking exercise may help to control IR and give a stronger repair – but if the horse becomes more lame when walking, or is worse the day after, this generally indicates that further mechanical breakdown is occurring, and the horse should be confined for longer, and its management reassessed.

It can be very difficult to get the correct

balance of 'as much exercise as possible without causing damage', but controlling the walking and any increase in exercise is far safer than just turning a horse out. The aim is to improve insulin sensitivity sufficiently to allow the laminar bonds to become stronger to cope with increased mechanical forces before they are subjected to them.

MEDICATION

It is important that any medication given to try to control IR is in conjunction with the necessary management changes of a low-sugar diet and exercise, rather than instead of them.

Metformin is one of the drugs used in man to control IR, and it does so by reducing glucose uptake from the gut and by improving insulin sensitivity. Studies indicate that Metformin is effective and safe in horses, but because it is poorly absorbed from the horse's intestines, its mode of action may be limited to blocking glucose uptake from the small intestine, thus reducing the insulin response to NSCs in the diet.

Thyroxine supplementation to IR horses is still common practice for horses in the USA. Thyroxine (T4) is produced in the thyroid gland, and its blood levels are often found to be low in insulin-resistant horses – but once IR is controlled, T4 returns to normal, so it is now generally considered to be as a result of IR, rather than a cause of it. Phenylbutazone (bute) lowers T4 production, and this may account for lower levels in some IR horses since testing may be done after they have developed laminitis. Thyroxine given to an obese horse does appear to help reduce the horse's weight by increasing its metabolic rate, and vets now tend to prescribe it for a limited period (possibly six months) until IR has been controlled by changes in the diet.

Horses should be 'weaned off' thyroxine by reducing the dosage, rather than stopping medication suddenly. Levothyroxine sodium (Thyro- L) is available in the USA and is relatively inexpensive, but the equivalent in the UK, Soloxine, which currently is what our 'drug cascade' requires us to use, is significantly more expensive.

CORTICOSTEROIDS

The possible role of corticosteroids in the development of IR has been discussed earlier in the chapter, with their likely effect being on glucose homeostasis and by directly inhibiting the action of insulin in tissues.

The risk of developing clinical laminitis following the administration of corticosteroids is widely reported, but probably occurs extremely rarely. There are certain factors that increase the risk, one being the length of action of the corticosteroid, and the long-acting synthetic corticosteroid Triamcinolone is recognized as a greater risk than short-acting steroids. Probably more important is if the patient receiving the injection is already insulin resistant. It seems likely that for some IR cases, corticosteroid medication is sufficient to worsen IR and tip the balance to cause the already weakened laminae to separate. Vets are aware of the potential risk of using corticosteroids, and every time they administer them have to weigh this up against the therapeutic benefits.

Increased corticosteroid release in response to chronic pain and stress can play a part in worsening IR and laminitis.

PPID

PPID (Pituitary Pars Intermedia Dysfunction, or Cushing's Disease, or Hyperadrenocorticism) is caused either by a growth in the pituitary gland at the base of the brain (pituitary adenoma), or by an enlargement of the gland (pituitary hyperplasia), and it is the middle part of the

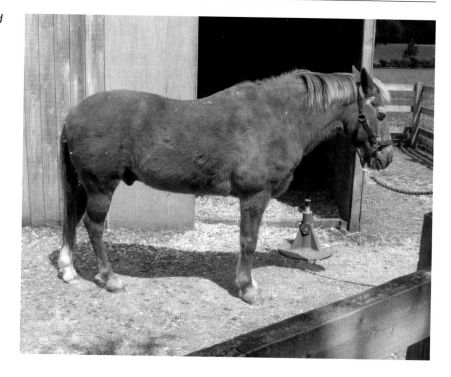

Fig. 158 A thirty-year-old pony with a thick coat in mid June (PPID).

pituitary gland, the pars intermedia, that is affected in the horse. It is characterized by increased hormone production from this part of the gland, including ACTH which, in turn, causes the adrenal gland to produce more corticosteroids.

The symptoms of PPID include the following:

- Hirsuitism – dense coat
- Insulin resistance
- Laminitis
- Weight loss
- Immunosuppression – persistent infections
- Polydipsia and polyuria
- Hyperhidrosis – excessive sweating
- Infertility

Some of the symptoms may be the result of other hormones produced by the affected pituitary gland, but many are due to the high levels of corticosteroids, and since PPID horses are often also insulin resistant, due to high levels of insulin.

PPID is a problem of the older horse and pony, generally over the age of fifteen years, but has been diagnosed in younger animals.

Hirsuitism, the most common symptom, is a change in the horse's coat. In the early stages this may be seen as abnormal seasonal shedding, progressing to a horse having an abnormally dense, curly coat in the later stages of the disease.

Horses with PPID can suffer weight loss, and if combined with insulin resistance can be thin while still having the fat deposits typical of IR.

Laminitis is a common problem of PPID, and if laminitis occurs with no obvious reason, or in cases that are slow to respond, the horse should be tested for IR and PPID.

Diagnosis

This can very often be made purely from the abnormal shedding of, or other changes in, the horse's coat, particularly if combined with some of the other symptoms, with studies suggesting that up to 85 per cent of PPID cases have these changes.

(It should be pointed out here that many of the symptoms we see in cases that are IR are also present in Cushing's disease (PPID). Part of the reason for this is that many of these PPID cases are also insulin resistant, but for these, if only the IR is addressed, the clinical problems are likely to continue until treatment is given for the PPID, and vice versa.)

Blood Tests

Horses with PPID will often have high blood insulin, but to differentiate from IR, blood can be taken to test for levels of ACTH, the current test of choice, or by using the Dexamethasone Suppression Test (DST).

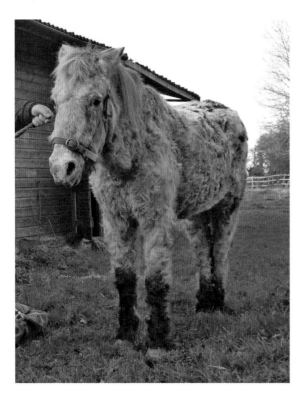

Fig. 159   A pony with untreated PPID, with IR and laminitis.

Samples to test for ACTH need to be taken into chilled tubes, frozen rapidly and sent frozen to the laboratory, which can cause practical problems 'in the field', and the DST involves testing the response to an injection of the corticosteroid dexamethasone, and therefore poses a potential risk to horses that are IR. Seasonal hormonal variation can make interpretation of the results from both of these tests more difficult when horses are tested in the autumn. Some labs have managed to redefine what is normal for samples taken in August, September and October, to account for the natural seasonal rise in ACTH, and because PPID horses tend to have dramatic rises in the autumn, these labs now suggest it as a good time to test.

ACTH levels can be raised in other circumstances, particularly when a horse is stressed, so it is recommended that the horse has blood taken when it is quiet and calm in its own environment. It must also be borne in mind that if tested during a bout of laminitis, a rise in ACTH may be due to the stress caused by pain, rather than from PPID.

Treatment

Pergolide is the most effective drug available, but there is some disagreement on what dose should be given. In many cases, 0.5–1mg will be given initially, with the dose raised depending on the response (possibly even up to 5mg, or more). Even when a low dose is apparently controlling the PPID, a higher dose may be required in the autumn when there is the 'seasonal rise' in ACTH production.

Cyproheptadine and chaste tree berry are sometimes given, and although they improve some of the symptoms of PPID, their effect appears to be limited.

Concomitant IR needs to be addressed with suitable dietary changes and, where possible, exercise.

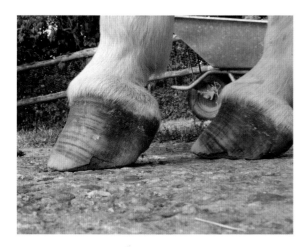

Fig. 160   A donkey with chronic foot changes. There are obvious growth rings, which diverge towards the heel in the right foot (on the right of the picture), accompanied by deviation in the line of the dorsal wall.

Because PPID horses are likely to have reduced defences (immuno-suppressed), they may require treatment for chronic infections. (They should be regularly wormed and vaccinated.)

IR AND LAMINITIS IN DONKEYS

A lack of exercise combined with constant access to pasture has resulted in a population of donkeys in the UK that are insulin resistant. Over three-quarters of the donkeys 'rescued' by sanctuaries in the UK have foot problems as a result of this.

Their foot problems are commonly the result of chronic changes from weakened laminae due to IR, which will, in most cases, produce insidious low-grade foot changes rather than be seen as obvious acute laminitis. This will partly be due to their sedentary life-style, which limits the mechanical forces acting on the feet, and partly due to their stoical nature, so that

early changes are less likely to be noticed. As a consequence of this, breakdown and widening of the white line, whether from acute or the more chronic laminitic changes, allows dirt to penetrate up the wall, and leads to the common problem in donkey feet of 'seedy toe'.

The growth rings around the hoof are often obvious and may diverge towards the heel, and there may be bends in the dorsal wall. When growth of the dorsal wall is slowed and the heels grow faster, the side walls usually remain upright. Donkeys are much less likely to respond to chronic pain with contracture of the

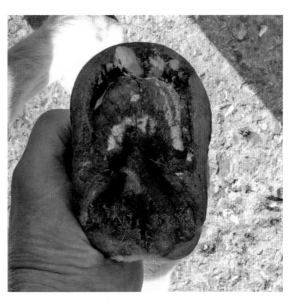

Fig. 161   The left fore of the donkey shown in Fig. 160. It was this foot that was causing lameness on this occasion, as a result of dirt and infection under the dorsal wall, through a chronically damaged 'white line' ('seedy toe').

deep flexor muscle, as occurs with small ponies that have similar chronic problems, and if the heels continue to grow faster, donkeys may stand and walk on the heels, with the heel wall in contact with the ground and the toe raised up off it (Fig. 162).

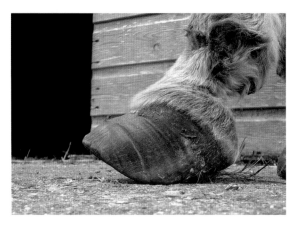

Fig. 162   A donkey with chronic laminitis standing on the hoof wall of an overgrown heel. (It also walked this way.)

Management

How to deal with donkeys that have feet with these chronic changes is a major problem, and is often what leads owners to give up and hand them over to rescue centres and donkey sanctuaries.

One thing is certain, and that is the donkey's insulin resistance has to be addressed before there is any chance of the foot problems being resolved satisfactorily. This generally has to rely on strict management of their diet, since controlled exercise is difficult to achieve, even with hand-walking, since many donkeys are extremely reluctant to be halter-led.

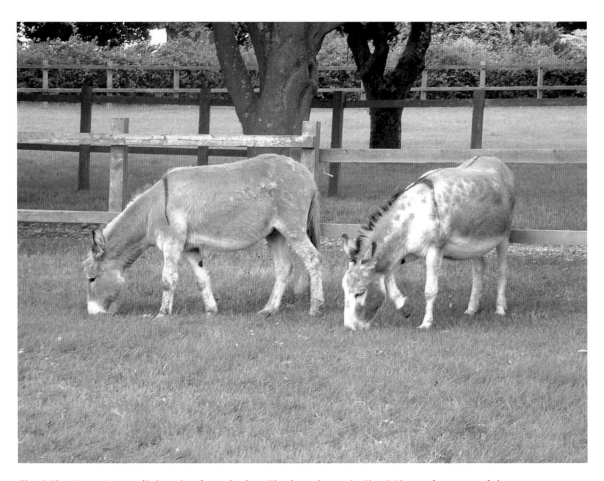

Fig. 163   Not a 'natural' situation for a donkey. The foot shown in Fig. 162 was from one of these.

Keeping donkeys off grass, or even limiting access to it (by time and/or muzzling) causes a problem for many owners since they have often acquired them to be companion animals for other horses, or to actually keep pastures under control. They no longer become the easy-to-manage and cheap-to-feed animals they were meant to be. If the donkey needs to be taken off grass, it is important that food is not restricted too much, since donkeys are prone to developing hyperlipidaemia if starved, and sufficient low-sugar, high-fibre food should be available.

It can be difficult to correct the foot problems, or even keep them under control, with seedy toe and recurrent foot abscesses presenting a real challenge. Using the dorsal wall angle as the indicator of how much heel to take off often results in farriers leaving P3 tilted excessively. This is particularly when there is little deviation in the dorsal wall and separation has occurred with rotation of P3 away from it, and because farriers have been told that donkey feet are more upright than those of horses, the heels are often left too long and the bone is left sharply angled down on to its tip. Radiography is extremely useful for providing information about what is going on in the feet, and this will help with their management.

9 Foot Problems with Visible Changes

HOOF CHANGES

The strength of the formed hoof wall makes it resistant to damage from the outside, so most problems involving the hoof structure result either from factors that affect its growth at the coronary band, or from damage at the ground-bearing surface.

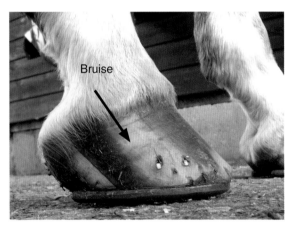

Fig. 164   'Bruises' can be seen on unpigmented hooves, but are not visible when the wall is pigmented.

Bruising

Reddened areas are commonly seen on the wall of unpigmented hooves. This appears to result from bruising at the coronary band, with the blood pigments growing down

with the wall, rather than coming from the laminae locally. These 'bruises' may be hidden by the periople, thus not visible in the upper part of the wall, nor will they be seen if the hoof is pigmented. Most commonly these bruises are localized, but they can be more widespread following obvious traumatic injury to the coronet or pastern, or as a strip of bruising growing down from the dorsal wall, such as accompanies laminitis. These large areas of bruising are recognized as symptoms of problems that presumably will already be receiving treatment, whereas more localized bruises usually occur without

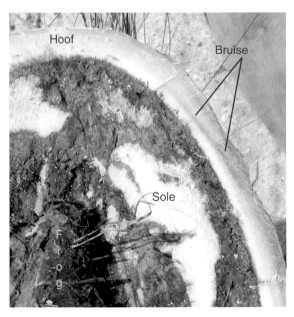

Fig.   165 More widespread bruising, but still restricted to the outer part of the wall.

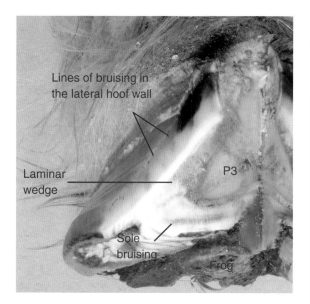

Fig. 166 *The cut lateral wall of a foot from a chronic laminitic horse (PPID and IR) with lines of bruising through the lateral wall. These accompanied probably minor episodes of laminitis, with the changes occurring along the length of the coronary groove and growing down from it. There are no blood pigments in the inner hoof wall. The sole bruising will also have occurred as a result of laminitis.*

commonly referred to as 'grass rings', but in other circumstances they may be called 'fever rings' or 'laminitis rings'.

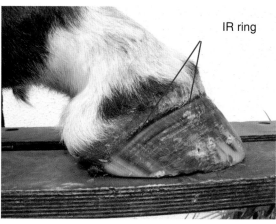

Fig. 167 *A hind foot (cadaver) with one obvious IR ring.*

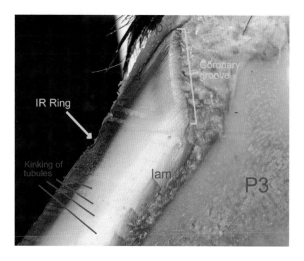

Fig. 168 *The same foot as in Fig. 167 cut midline showing kinks in the tubules, through the different strata, at different levels down the wall. The tubules were affected at the same point of growth but started off lower down the wall because of the shape of the coronary groove (see also Fig. 143). Each area through the wall where there is kinking of the tubules has straight tubules attached on each side, helping affected hoof wall to maintain its strength.*
Key: *P = periople, lam = the laminae*

any apparent lameness, and only become evident lower down the wall several months later, to eventually grow out with the wall at the ground surface.

A common place for bruises to appear is at the toe quarter, and it is possible that they are the result of bruising at the coronary band from stresses on the distal wall below it. All there is to do for these, and similar bruises, is to try to make sure the foot is balanced to remove areas of stress on the wall.

IR Rings (Grass Rings, Laminitis Rings or Fever Rings)

In some circumstances growth rings around the foot are more obvious, often being attributed to changes in nutrition; in the UK these are

These obvious rings are slight indentations on the hoof surface, and they develop at the coronary band from a change in growth at the top of the hoof wall. What causes this kink on the outer surface affects the growth, simultaneously, along the length of the coronary groove. Fig. 168 (and Fig. 143) shows kinking of the tubules through the thickness of the hoof wall, but in a lower position down the wall than the outer hoof ring, mirroring the shape of the coronary groove. Sometimes an obvious ring will appear in a single hoof when injury, infection or swelling affects hoof growth in that foot, but more commonly all four feet are affected. When this occurs, the cause of these obvious rings is from some systemic change, sometimes as a result of an alteration in diet or from an inflammatory, toxic or metabolic condition.

break in growth of the intertubular horn, similar to that seen in sole and frog growth. For the sole and frog, as the superficial layer dries out, the weak point in the intertubular horn breaks down, after which the tubules from the layer underneath, which are still embedded in the outer layer, break off so that the outer layer can be shed. The hoof remains intact as it grows down, but the growth rings still represent a weak point which is exploited by other factors affecting hoof growth, and this can cause the tubules to kink, and produce indentations and ridges in the wall. Through the thickness of the wall, the bending in the horn tubules through the different layers is adjacent and firmly attached to tubular and intertubular horn that grew down from the coronary band at a different time, in a slightly different growth cycle. These adjacent tubules provide support to the ones that are bent, and limit the amount they kink.

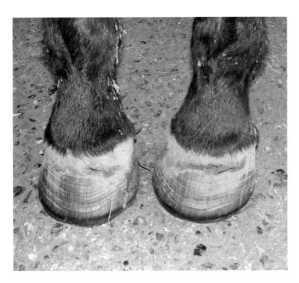

Fig. 169   The front feet of a Warmblood × Show pony, showing matching rings around the them, which were also present on the hind feet.

What do the obvious Growth Rings represent?

The regular faint growth rings on the normal hoof appear to indicate an intermittent

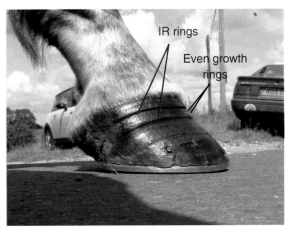

Fig. 170   In between the two obvious IR rings, there have been three growth cycles, with two evenly spaced growth lines. It is quite likely that this horse's IR was still not under control after the lower of the two rings appeared (where the hoof deviation occurs), but the effect of the forces up the wall acted on the already bent tubules rather than the new growth, allowing them to grow down apparently normally, with the IR ring becoming deeper and more obvious.

When a horse develops laminitis, not only do the laminae start to separate but the coronary attachment is also affected, and the new growth of horn that is produced directly after this, grows down with a very obvious ring, indicating when the separation occurred; moreover this is very often accompanied by deviation of the wall at this site. I think that 'grass rings' represent changes in growth similar to this, but where the integrity of the wall has been maintained sufficiently for no clinical signs of lameness to be seen.

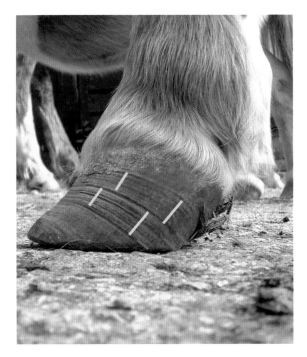

Fig. 171 Pony with chronic laminitis, where most growth rings are accentuated on the dorsal wall, appearing as indentations and ridges. The rings diverge towards the heel.

Because these obvious rings are so common in the population of horses and ponies considered at risk of developing laminitis, as well as those that do develop it, I believe they are related to IR and represent low-grade laminitis. They appear following changes in the grass, because this has affected the horse's control of its IR, and caused weakening of the connection and kinking of the tubules, and this is why I prefer to call them 'IR rings'.

Why do IR Rings Occur?

IR rings would seem to occur due to the effect of forces on new horn growth coinciding with the break between growth cycles, causing the tubules to kink as they are formed. How much of an indentation occurs depends on the extent of weakening, and of the forces acting on the hoof. In Fig. 170, continuing mechanical forces up the wall were concentrated on the already bent tubules, and this allowed the new wall above it to grow down straight over the next three cycles. When this IR ring became stabilized, continued IR weakening and mechanical forces on the wall affected the new growth to produce a second IR ring above it. In cases when wall-weakening is greater, the mechanical forces on the wall cause laminar detachment, and the low-grade laminitis progresses to clinical laminitis.

The feet of chronic laminitics have less support from the dorsal wall due to the damaged laminar attachment, and sometimes nearly every growth ring can be exaggerated (Fig. 171). I have suggested previously that the divergent growth rings occurring around the hooves in these cases are due to slowed hoof growth of the dorsal wall from pressure on the coronary blood supply; however, part of the difference may be due to the tubules kinking, which reduces the distance between the rings and shortens hoof length.

Not all the obvious rings round the hoof are due to IR or laminitis. If the rings follow some form of systemic infection or toxic condition, the horse is more likely to have a single deep

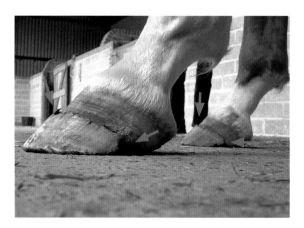

Fig. 172   This Thoroughbred yearling lived out in a field, without any apparent problem, until it went lame on one front foot. Something must have happened to this horse about five months earlier to have caused hoof growth to stop briefly (the reason was not known). The dorsal wall of all four feet separated at the same position, with the more distal part still attached to the laminae (these are the two hind feet). The lameness was caused by the laminae at the defect being pinched by the movement of the partially attached hoof. The proximal hoof grew down normally.

ring, evident on all four feet, and the term 'fever rings' might be used to describe them. Sometimes these will be particularly severe, and although the hoof grows down with the defect, it is only when the heel grows out at the ground and the rest of the wall loses its support that it becomes evident that growth actually stopped for a time, enough for the upper and lower portion of the hoof to separate and become unstable (*see* Fig. 172).

Obvious growth rings can occur in one foot when its coronary circulation is affected, possibly from an injury to the pastern or coronet, or following an infection, when the leg swells dramatically, as in lymphangitis.

In the absence of another cause, horses with obvious growth rings on their feet need to be assessed for IR, and if this seems likely, the diet should be changed and exercise should be increased in a controlled way, to allow strengthening of the laminae.

Wounds of the Pastern and Heel

Disruption to the coronary blood supply due to swelling resulting from pastern injuries will often result in exaggerated growth rings on the hoof, and non-pigmented feet may also have 'bruising' as blood products from the wound are incorporated into new horn growth. Far more of a problem is when a pastern wound also involves the coronary band. Most commonly this will be from wounds from direct trauma, from 'over-reaching' by a hind foot, and from rope or wire injuries.

The decision whether or not to suture a pastern wound will depend on its size, position, and the degree of tissue damage that has been caused by the trauma: thus cuts will generally be sutured, but deep rope burns will probably not be, since the damaged tissues are very unlikely to hold the sutures. All pastern wounds involving the coronary band should be sutured, if at all possible, to try to get the coronary band to heal with the least distortion, in order to limit scarring and the abnormal hoof growth that will subsequently grow down from this.

The nature of the injuries and the amount of tissue movement often cause wounds of the heel bulbs to break down if sutured, so this type of wound will often be left to heal by second intention (allowed to heal 'naturally'). If this is the case, the defect fills with granulation tissue to bind the two sides of the wound together. Healing and resolution of the problem generally takes about six weeks, although the horse will often be sound a couple of weeks before this. Problems can occur if the granulation tissue proliferates (often referred to as 'proud flesh'), leading to delayed healing, and it may leave significant scarring on the heel bulb. Applying a plaster cast to a sutured heel-bulb wound can reduce the chances of wound breakdown by limiting movement of the tissues and by providing support and protection.

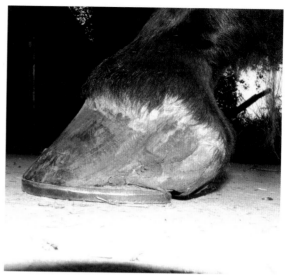

Fig. 174   Hoof growth from a scarred and distorted coronary band can look ugly but often does not cause a problem. However, it is more likely to do so if the horse is shod very short at the heel, as in this case.

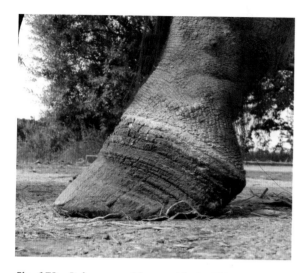

Fig. 173   Polo pony with sarcoidosis. This seemed to be localized to below the left hind hock in this case.

Other Conditions affecting the Pastern

Some conditions that affect the pastern can produce hoof changes. Inflammation caused by '**Mud Fever**' may cause the periople to become thicker and roughened. The severe oedema caused by **Lymphangitis** can affect hoof growth, when an obvious ring around the wall is produced. Lymphangitis occurs when an infectious focus in a leg affects the lymphatics, limiting fluid drainage and resulting in a very swollen leg, two or even three times its normal size. **Sarcoidosis** is a rare condition that can cause severe crusting of the skin that can be localized or widespread. When this occurs on the pastern, obvious changes will be seen in the hoof.

Other organs in the body can be affected by this condition and can result in severe wasting.

Hoof Scars

If an injured coronary band heals with scarring and distortion, abnormal horn will be permanently produced from it. Sometimes these scars and the distorted hoof can look very unsightly, but with good hoof care, many cases do not cause a problem. The most common problems that do occur with these are from the development of hoof cracks, and from poor connection to the sole at the ground surface, which leaves the feet more prone to white line disease and local abscesses.

Quittor

Quittor refers to an infection involving a collateral cartilage, generally following a wound to the pastern and coronary band, and causes a persistent discharge from part of the wound once the remainder has healed. This generally requires surgery to remove infected and necrotic (dead) cartilage, otherwise this continues to act as a 'foreign body' and the problem persists.

HOOF CRACKS

If the laminae are intact, the hoof can generally withstand the forces that act on it by spreading the load; however, if the forces are constantly uneven, they can cause the hoof to bend and distort, and if the stress is more concentrated it may cause a split or crack to develop. Superficial cracks of the more rigid, tubule-dense outer wall follow the line of the tubules, but are generally prevented from spreading through the thickness of the wall by the greater suppleness of the moister inner wall and the characteristics of the intertubular horn.

Horizontal Cracks

Horizontal cracks rarely occur from direct trauma to the hoof, and in most cases grow down in the wall as a result of a temporary interruption of growth after damage to the coronary band. Very many of these result from hoof abscesses that have tracked up the wall and burst out at the coronary band, but occasionally they occur when a foot strikes a solid object such as a tree stump with sufficient force, or hits something solid when kicking out; these are sometimes accompanied by a fracture of P3. New hoof produced above any horizontal crack will generally grow down normally.

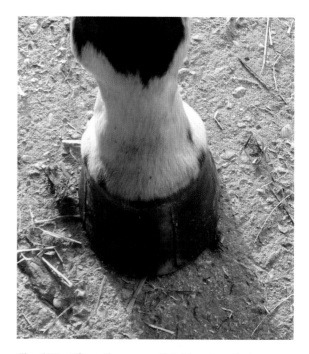

Fig. 175 These three superficial hoof cracks have become more obvious due to repeated wetting and drying of the hoof (the environmental conditions).

Vertical Hoof Cracks

Superficial Cracks

Superficial cracks generally result from minor damage to the coronary band, and grow out with the hoof once the injury settles. However, they will grow down constantly if the coronet heals with a small defect. These are generally of little consequence, although they do represent a weakness in the wall which greater forces can take advantage of, and occasionally a superficial crack can spread to involve the deeper layers.

Full Thickness Cracks

Cracks from the ground surface include the following:

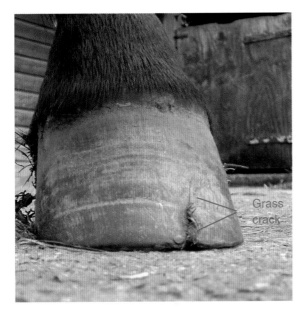

Fig. 176 A 'grass crack' in a yearling's foot. This can allow dirt and infection to reach the sensitive structures.

a) **Grass cracks:** When the foot becomes overgrown and the wall extends beyond the level of the sole, the hoof is less able to maintain a uniform shape and may flare, split or break away. Cracks starting at the ground surface may not reach the sensitive structures, but at other times will do so directly, or may allow dirt and infection to access these deeper tissues.

b) **Heel cracks:** The heel quarter is an area that is often overloaded, being the site of a fold in the hoof when a heel loses its support and turns under, and cracks can develop here.

c) **Bar cracks:** These most often occur where the bar joins the sole on its anterior border.

When overgrown, distortion of the bars can produce uneven forces on this junction, and although many of these cracks are superficial, occasionally they can involve the full thickness.

d) **Sandcracks:** These cracks start at the coronary band, they involve the full thickness of the wall, and are classified by their position, with toe and quarter cracks being the most common.

Quarter cracks appear to develop as the result of internal forces at the heel quarters. The position of these cracks is usually slightly more dorsal (anterior) than those starting from the ground as a result of heel collapse. When the limb is weighted and the pastern drops, the distal (lower) end of P2 forces the collateral cartilages out and puts pressure on the wall at the quarters. A higher position of the wall relative to the internal structures – for example, with a sheared heel – increases the force on it from the collateral cartilage. It is suggested that an average size foot with less than 15mm cartilage palpable above the wall is more prone to developing a quarter crack.

Toe cracks develop in the midline and appear to be caused by abnormal forces part way down the wall. I described in Chapter 4 how the dorsal wall of medium-strength feet can, in some cases, bend inwards in the upper part of the hoof, and it seems that the forces that produce this can also cause a split to develop. These cracks appear to start between a third and half way down the wall, at the depth of the bend, and then spread up to involve the coronary band. The initial split follows the line of the tubules, but as it works upwards, the more hydrated upper wall tries to deflect it transversely along the layers of intertubular horn, producing a defect at the coronary band which is often kinked rather than straight, while the wall defect below the crack may remain superficial.

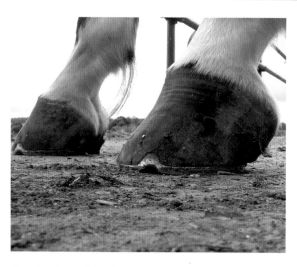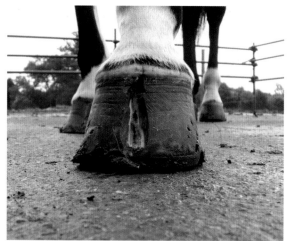

Figs. 177a and 177b   This foot originally had a superficial crack on the dorsal wall, and this was one occasion where it progressed to being a deep crack, due to the way the foot was trimmed and shod. The dorsal wall is being forced inward as a result of the foot's long toe and upright heels.

Hoof cracks that penetrate through to the sensitive dermis cause pain, particularly when the horse moves, as the two sides move independently of each other, causing stretching or pinching of the laminae. Toe cracks will generally close up as the foot is weighted, and widen when the foot is lifted off the ground, but quarter cracks are more likely to open up when the foot is weighted. Cracks also provide a means of entry for infection through to the sensitive dermis.

Treatment of Hoof Cracks

Farriers often groove or burn the wall above a ground crack, or try to isolate a sandcrack by making a 'V' groove starting below the defect to try to prevent it spreading. Full thickness cracks require more aggressive action. The two main aims are to reduce the forces on the wall that caused the split, and to stabilize the two sides of the crack to allow new, intact growth to occur – but other factors such as poor horn quality may also need to be addressed.

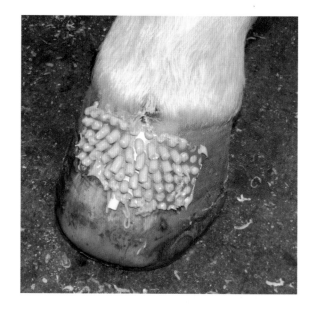

Fig. 178   This foot had a 'toe crack' similar to that shown in Fig. 177. A straw was placed in the depth of the crack before Bond-n-Flex and a perforated aluminium plate were applied. The straw was then removed and this allowed the crack to be flushed. The Bond-n-Flex was smoothed off. This application provided stability to the wall for the crack to grow out. (This method was also used successfully with the foot in Fig. 180.)

The foot should be balanced to reduce uneven forces, and cracks starting from the ground surface will benefit from any overgrown wall being trimmed. When dealing with a quarter crack the foot needs to be trimmed to reduce the torsion on it from uneven landing, and to address sheared heels when these are present. Toe cracks tend to occur in feet that have restricted movement of the heels accompanied by a long toe. The forces on the dorsal wall need to be reduced by easing breakover, but heel movement also needs to be facilitated, either by reducing heel height or, if this is not possible or desirable, by trimming the bars to a greater extent.

The crack needs to be cleaned out before stabilizing the two sides, and farriers have different ways of dealing with this. Some use screws and wires, or a metal plate screwed to the wall (a Nolan plate) or fixed with hoof filler, and if shoes are put on there may be some change in clip placement. If the wall is stabilized and the underlying cause addressed, the hoof will usually grow down attached, and the problem resolves.

PROBLEMS OF THE BEARING SURFACE

Thrush

'Thrush' is an infection involving the frog, and often affecting the central and collateral sulci, but it can become more widespread to involve the body of the frog. It is characterized by a black discharge and a very unpleasant smell. Lameness due to thrush may be worse on soft ground when there is greater ground contact with the frog, but sometimes it is only detected when cleaning the clefts out with the hoofpick, from sensitivity or bleeding. Horses with deep clefts in their frogs stabled on soiled bedding will be more prone to thrush, particularly if the feet are not regularly picked out, since this provides conditions for anaerobic bacteria to proliferate.

A variety of organisms may be involved, with the anaerobic bacterium *Fusobacterium necrophorus* being the most widely mentioned, while some organisms involved are keratolytic, and have the ability to degrade the frog horn.

Management and Treatment

The aim is to trim away any damaged frog to allow effective antibacterial and antifungal treatment of infected tissue, and by exposing this, air will help to control any anaerobic bacteria that are involved. Horses that are stabled a lot should be kept in clean conditions and have their feet picked out regularly. Exercise is recommended since this improves circulation and will help with normal frog exfoliation.

Partial shedding of frog layers is a normal process, and although removal of loose pieces will avoid pockets where infection can start, excessive trimming should be avoided as removal of the hardened superficial layer will initially leave the softer, deeper layers less well protected, more sensitive on uneven and stony ground, and more liable to damage.

If the feet are soaked or poulticed, it is normal for the wetness to pick up any dirt, to produce a blackened liquid, but this should not be confused with the discharge produced in thrush (identified by its foul smell). As with the sole, degeneration of the frog horn between the more superficial layers before shedding, can sometimes be white and powdery, and this is unlikely to be due to a 'fungal infection' as some suggest.

There are a large number of proprietary antibacterial and antifungal products marketed for the treatment of thrush, and intramammary antibiotic preparations, metronidazole paste, hydrogen peroxide, oxine, acid cider vinegar, and iodine preparations are sometimes used.

'Canker' (Hypertrophic pododermatitis)

Canker is a particularly unpleasant proliferative disease involving the frog, and often spreads to involve tissues around it. Finger-like papillae grow from the affected tissue, and these bleed easily. Rather than having a primary infectious agent that causes canker, there is now some evidence that canker has a similar pathogenesis to sarcoids that develop in the skin, which may account for the way the condition progresses and the difficulty in treating it.

It is not a common condition, and it seems to occur extremely rarely in the UK. It is reported to be seen most commonly in draft horses kept in dirty conditions. Treatment involves extensive surgery to remove all the affected tissue, but canker very often recurs. It has been reported that the frequency of this is reduced if surgery is followed up with topical chemotherapy (Cisplatin, which is only suitable for use in a veterinary hospital).

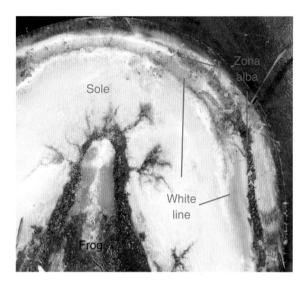

Fig. 179   WLD affecting the unpigmented hoof ('zona alba') of a pony foot, and dirt pressing into the defect has displaced the 'white line'.

'White Line' Disease (WLD)

The confusion about what to call the 'white line' continues, because 'white line disease' (WLD) is used, in different literature, to refer to both disease of the 'white line' as well as disease of the unpigmented hoof wall outside it.

WLD Affecting the Wall

Although we see erosion of the unpigmented hoof, it would appear to be less of a problem in the UK than in the USA, where it seems more commonly to cause large areas of horn erosion right up the wall. This could be due to different bacteria or fungi involved, different environmental conditions (humidity), or different diet. Fungi that destroy keratin (keratolytic) have been isolated from some cases, and these thrive on this damaged horn.

It may be that it is noticed sooner here in the UK because dirt and mud pack up into the cavity to produce lameness at an earlier stage. Without this dirt getting in, this type of WLD is often not a painful problem until it progresses to where the stability of the hoof is compromised.

WLD Involving the 'White Line'

The 'white line' can lose its integrity when erosion occurs from outside, or from abnormal formation of 'white line' horn from the inside, from distortion of the terminal papillae following separation of the laminae in laminitis. In post-laminitis cases, the 'white line' is wider and weaker, making it more liable to split and thereby allowing dirt and infection to gain entry. (*See* 'Abscesses' in Chapter 11.)

'White line' horn quality is affected by the ground and environmental conditions it has to deal with, but also by the horse's diet, which affects how it is able to deal with these conditions.

Nutrition and Horn Growth

Balancing a horse's diet, based on its age and lifestyle, is important for its overall health as well as the condition of its hooves, and the effects of dietary deficiencies or excesses will often first be noticed by the way the hoof and 'white line' fail to cope. In fact the effects of changes of nutrition on horn growth will be seen at the ground surface much sooner in the 'white line' (even as early as six weeks), as opposed to the nine months it takes the dorsal wall to grow down to the ground.

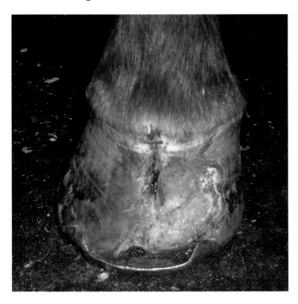

Fig. 180   Extensive WLD of the unpigmented wall ('zona alba')destabilized the hoof, and combined with poor trimming/shoeing, led to the midline 'toe crack' developing.

A horse's diet should contain adequate **protein**, but if this is low, poor hooves will only be one symptom of an unthrifty animal. Fats are needed in the diet to produce the lipids that are involved in cell-to-cell adhesion and

for producing a permeability barrier that helps prevent bacterial and fungal penetration of the horn.

Nearly thirty years ago it was suggested that supplementation of **biotin** (one of the B vitamins) improved the condition of horses' hooves. However, theoretically horses should obtain all the biotin they need, since it is produced by bacteria in the hind gut, and it has been found that only a small percentage of horses with poor feet showed any improvement as a result of the supplementary feeding of biotin; moreover this would often be in horses under working stress or fed low quality diets.

A low **calcium/phosphorus** (Ca:P) ratio in a horse's diet can affect calcium's involvement in the formation of firm attachments between keratinocytes. High levels of phosphorus in a diet block calcium absorption, resulting in crumbling horn because of weaker cellular attachments, affecting particularly the inner layers of the hoof and the 'white line'. Bran in particular has a very low Ca:P ratio (lower calcium and higher phosphorus), and horses stabled on a grain and bran diet with hay will commonly have weak feet that have difficulty retaining shoes. A good way to improve the Ca:P in the diet is to stop the bran, reduce the grain, and introduce some alfalfa into the diet, since this has high levels of protein and calcium, and a low phosphorus content. Diets with a ratio of less than 1:1 are likely to produce the problem, and a ratio of around 1.6 Ca:1.0 P is recommended.

Methionine is included in many 'hoof supplements', this amino acid being important in the disulfide bond formation that gives keratin its strength. Balanced diets with 10–12 per cent protein levels are thought likely to contain sufficient methionine, but supplementation may be necessary in some cases. However, over-supplementation of methionine causes degeneration of the 'white line', by affecting the inter-tubular horn while leaving the tubules intact, and this then spreads outwards through the hoof layers, the effect being attributed to a zinc deficiency. Methionine binds easily with zinc to increase its absorption (it decreases copper absorption), but in high doses, this ease of binding may cause excessive excretion of zinc to produce a deficiency. The problem is corrected, in most cases, by stopping methionine supplementation.

Selenium is necessary for muscle development, and after the suggestion that it helped to prevent recurrence of azoturia ('tying-up'), selenium supplementation became very popular. However, it is very important not to over-supplement selenium because of its effect on keratin production. By replacing sulfur, excess selenium limits the formation of strong disulfide bonds, which results in weaker horn being produced. In acute selenium poisoning, weak horn production around the whole

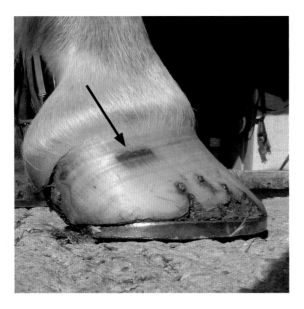

Fig. 181 Under-running hoof wall degradation associated with infection around the nail holes. The blackness is the result of sulfur-reducing bacteria reacting with the shoe nails. This foot had an abscess involving these bacteria, which broke out at the coronary band. The horizontal crack has grown down the wall (arrow) with discoloration from the infection in the hoof wall below it.

coronary band is one possible cause of the separation seen in Fig. 172.

Carbohydrates are an integral part of the diet, but the effect of high NSC in the diet has been discussed in Chapter 8.

The effect of environmental factors on poor quality horn is much greater than for normal horn. Affected feet are more likely to deteriorate if they are constantly wet or kept on soiled bedding, with increased degradation from faeces and from ammonia produced by the breakdown of urine. Bacterial involvement in WLD appears to be secondary to impaired horn production, in many cases with proliferation of anaerobic bacteria (these thrive in the absence of oxygen), but some of these, and some fungi, are particularly good at perpetuating the problem by actively breaking down keratin. Exposing the affected tissues to air and removing infected tissue can produce dramatic improvements, but some cases require hoof disinfectants in order to be fully resolved.

The treatment and control of WLD depends on the following factors:

- providing a balanced diet
- regular foot trimming to reduce the mechanical forces
- removing infected horn
- improving the foot environment
- treating the area with a suitable topical disinfectant

Seedy Toe and Wall Separation

Seedy toe can be a consequence of either forms of WLD. Whether a cavity is produced by degradation of the unpigmented wall or of the 'white line' following laminitis, it can be filled with dirt, which can enlarge the affected area by physical separation. Pain is generally caused by the pressure of dirt pushing up between the hoof and the sensitive laminae, rather than directly from any infection, since in both cases the sensitive dermis will still be protected by a keratinous layer (Figs 180 and 203).

Seedy toe is a very common problem in donkey feet because of the high incidence of insulin resistance in the UK donkey population, with changes to the laminae and 'white line' as a consequence of this.

Dealing with Wall Separation and Seedy Toe

The large cavity produced by WLD is only likely to settle down if the defect is fully exposed and the infected tissue is removed, back to healthy horn. Because the underlying cause of seedy toe can be due to IR and chronic laminitis, the decision whether to remove the overlying wall will depend on the stability of the bone and whether IR is under control. Depending on the extent of the cavity, some external means of stabilizing the hoof may be required, which may be provided by a hoof cast or a shoe. In

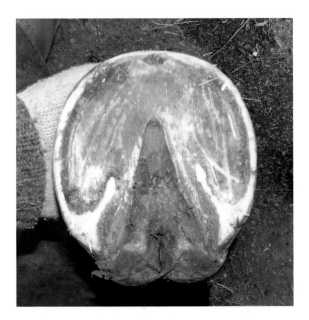

Fig. 182   The 'white line' at the tip of the toe is a common place to have a small local area of separation where dirt will collect – a 'black hole'.

cases where large sections of wall are removed, shoes can help provide a base for hoof-filler application and protection where it joins to the sole, but nail holes can further weaken compromised wall.

The 'Black Hole'

Not uncommonly a localized area of WLD occurs at the toe, mentioned not because of the problem it causes, but because of the frequency with which it is seen, and because dirt collects there. It has been given the sinister title 'the black hole' (K.C. la Pierre). A number of features often seem to occur together, and this makes it difficult to work out which of them initiates the situation.

It seems to occur in feet that are stressed at the toe; most commonly it is a problem of flatter, more spread feet, but it is also recognized in feet that are too upright.

The crena of P3 (*crena marginis solearis*) is a notch in the solar border of the bone at the toe, often seen on radiographs, frequently enough not to be considered abnormal. This may be a vestigial notch, since this was present in the bones of the horse's ancestors.

Casts of the blood vessels of a foot will sometimes have an indent in the circumflex blood vessels that run around the perimeter of the foot.

Above where the dirt collects there is often a conical-shaped zone of dense horn.

It occurs in both shod horses and those that have never had a shoe on, which tends to rule out the toe clip on the shoe as being the cause, although it still could contribute to it.

Very often these do not seem to cause a problem, with the dense horn providing protection and limiting the spread, but occasionally they can be the starting point for more extensive wall separation or seedy toe. Trimming to reduce the stress at the toe is important, to try to avoid this.

Bruised Sole

A bruised sole can cause lameness, but external evidence of this will not be seen at the time. When the sole dermis is bruised, blood is incorporated into the growing sole and grows down with it until it becomes evident on the ground surface six to eight weeks later. Not uncommonly, reddened areas are found on the sole when the surface is pared away, without having apparently caused lameness. Sole bruising may be caused by:

- external damage from stones or uneven ground
- prominent areas of retained sole
- the sole having been taken down too low, causing bruising of the terminal papillae around the white line
- episodes of laminitis, after which areas of bruising from under the tip of P3 may be found (*see* Figs 166 and 204)

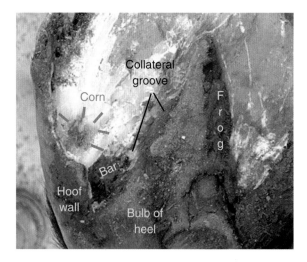

Fig. 183   'Corn' in the lateral heel of the right fore of a Thoroughbred. The flattened bar and turned-under heel have been cut away to take pressure off and expose the bruise.

Corns

The 'seat of corn' is the area of sole between the bar and the heel wall, and a bruise in this area is referred to as a 'corn'.

Corns are particularly a problem in shod horses with collapsed heels. When the wall folds under and the bars become curved, pressure is put on to the seat of corn and when a shoe is fitted on top of this, bruising occurs. This is compounded if the horse is shod short, or the period between shoeing is too long, so that the ends of the shoe are no longer supported by the wall and press directly on to this area (Fig. 73). Corns are painful and cause lameness, with the horse taking a shorter stride to avoid putting pressure on the heel. Sometimes infection will gain entry to the compromised tissue to further complicate the situation.

For corns to settle down, pressure must be removed from the area, and the first step is to trim back the folded wall and bar. Whether a bar shoe, or a boot with a pad or an Equicast is used to treat this, it is important that no pressure is put on the area, to allow it to settle down.

10 Lameness Investigation

In cases where there is no indication of the site of pain – or where a site has been found but it needs to be pinpointed in order to achieve a diagnosis – there are several ways to investigate these further. Nerve blocks and radiography are the simplest and most commonly used of these, but investigations may also involve joint blocks, ultrasound, thermography, radio-isotope scintigraphy, computed tomography (CT scan) or the use of magnetic resonance imaging (MRI).

NERVE BLOCK

Properly known as 'regional nerve blockade', this procedure is most commonly referred to as 'nerve block' and involves the injection of local anaesthetic adjacent to a nerve (perineurally); this desensitizes (numbs) the tissues local to and distal to (below) the injection site. Many people will have had experience of this, when a dentist has numbed an area of their mouth to allow work to be carried out on their teeth without pain.

The most common use of nerve blocks in horses is as an aid to diagnosing lameness, but they can also be used to help treat injuries and to suture wounds of the distal limb. The aim is to numb a specific localized area, and if investigating a lame horse, to identify if this improves or completely removes the lameness. Injecting local anaesthetic close to the medial and lateral palmar digital nerves will reduce or remove the lameness if the pain is caused by a

problem in the foot, but will have no effect on lameness if this arises from damage higher up the limb, above the block.

Pain in the palmar third of the foot and sole is generally removed by blocking the nerves at the level of the pastern (low palmar digital nerve block), but pain elsewhere in the foot requires a further nerve block higher up the leg. To include the nerve branches of the rest of the foot, local anaesthetic is injected close to the nerves as they pass over the outside (abaxial surface) of the sesamoid bones; this is referred to as an 'abaxial-sesamoid' block.

JOINT BLOCK

A joint block involves the injection of local anaesthetic directly into a joint and is used to locate lameness due to pain involving a specific joint. This desensitizes the sensory nerves in the joint, so that if the horse goes sound directly following a joint block, it would indicate that lameness is due to a problem involving that joint.

The Use of Nerve and Joint Blocks

The following practical considerations should be observed when using nerve and joint blocks.

- Both nerve and joint blocks need to be carried out under strict aseptic conditions, so the site of injection needs to be clipped and thoroughly cleansed. A clean environment is important to achieve this, and vets will almost certainly refuse to carry out a blocking procedure if the horse is presented with the legs still covered in mud.

- Blocking of the lower nerve branches is carried out first, working up to the higher branches, until the horse becomes sound.
- As small a dose as possible of local anaesthetic is used to minimize tissue irritation at the injection site and to reduce spread of the anaesthetic to affect other nerve branches, which would make the block less specific.
- Diagnostic joint blocks can only be carried out once the effect of any previous nerve block has gone, and sensation has returned.

Nerve and joint blocks are relatively cheap and easy to do, but sometimes will be time-consuming if serial nerve blocks up the leg are required to localize the problem, and this will increase the cost.

Identification of the site of lameness can be complicated by variations in the anatomical position of the digital nerves. In addition to this, the identification of injured areas using MRI has demonstrated that previously considered diagnostic joint blocks, particularly of the coffin joint and the navicular bursa, can turn out to be not so specific. Nevertheless, even taking this into consideration, both nerve and joint blocks are likely to localize the source of pain sufficiently so that a further detailed examination of the suspected area can be made. Radiography is most commonly the next step taken.

RADIOGRAPHY

Radiography uses the property of x-rays to pass through an object to produce images of its internal structure on a film, or digital receptor, placed beyond the object:

- A radiograph is the image that is produced by the effect of x-rays on a film or digital receptor.
- X-rays make up a form of electromagnetic radiation of very small wavelength, about 10,000 times shorter than that of visible light.
- 'X-rayed' is commonly used instead of 'radiographed', and 'x-rays' used when referring to radiographs

The interpretation of radiographs takes experience, and an owner could not be expected to be able to diagnose a problem from a radiograph; however, some knowledge of how it is obtained should help them understand what they are looking at if they are presented with one.

X-rays and the Production of Radiographs

For medical investigation, the x-rays generated in an x-ray machine are directed as a beam towards the object being investigated, for instance the foot of the horse. X-rays pass through the different tissues to a varying degree, and radiographic film placed on the other side of the foot reacts to the x-rays that reach it. The film is enclosed in a cassette that contains intensifying screens that convert the energy of the x-ray beam into light (fluorescence). This fluorescence is picked up by the x-ray film, producing a latent image that does not become visible until the film is developed, similar to the negative of a photograph.

Silver compounds on radiographic film, when activated by x-rays, release black metallic silver, so that if the x-ray beam reaches the film without passing through any tissue, this area will be seen as black on the developed film. More dense parts of the foot, particularly the bones, absorb the greatest amounts of energy from the beam, which limits the x-rays reaching the film, and this area will appear white on the developed film, and tissues that are thinner or less dense will appear as varying shades of grey.

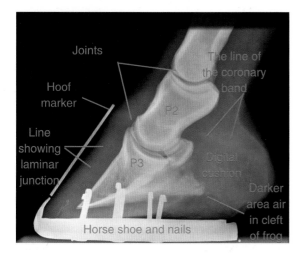

Fig. 184 A lateromedial radiograph. **Bright white:** *The metal shoe, nails and marker on the dorsal wall.* **White:** *The bones P1, P2, P3 and the navicular bone and areas of calcification of the collateral cartilages. The variation in shade is due to the density of the bone as well as the thickness that the x-rays pass through – the dense outer cortex and the less dense central medulla. Grey areas: The hoof wall is a lighter grey (denser) than the dermis between it and the coffin bone. Darker areas in the back part of the foot are the less dense digital cushion, and darker still is the air space in the collateral sulci of the frog. The line of the coronary band can be made out as it curves down towards the heel.*

If the output of x-rays from the machine is too high for the nature and thickness of tissue, an over-exposed film will be obtained that will be too dark to differentiate between structures; and if insufficient power is used, too few x-rays penetrate the tissues, which results in an under-exposed radiograph where everything is too white. The exposure and contrast of a radiograph will be affected by a number of factors: the type of x-rays generated, the strength of the beam, the distance between the source and the film, the nature and thickness of tissue being examined, the type of film and intensifying screen used (in a cassette), as well as the film development process.

The use of 'digital' radiography is now becoming more common, and with these, either the film in the cassette is converted to a digital image by a computer, or the x-ray beam is picked up directly on to a screen and converted to a digital image. These images can be manipulated in the same way as photographs can be manipulated on a computer, which as well as avoiding the problems involved in developing radiographic film, make it possible to produce radiographs of different contrast and definition from a single exposure. The end result is always a two-dimensional image of the structures of the foot.

RADIATION SAFETY

Radiation from x-rays is hazardous, and the dose must be kept to a minimum for both the horse and those in attendance. The following safety code should be observed.

- As few people as possible should be present, and those who are should wear protective lead-lined gowns.
- Pregnant women and children under the age of sixteen must leave the area.
- No part of an operator's or handler's body should be in the line of the primary x-ray beam.
- The spread of the beam should be limited to the area under investigation (collimation).
- The number of exposures should be kept to a minimum.

What are Radiographs Used For?

It is sometimes possible to identify pathological changes in the less dense structures, which is of particular importance in cases of laminitis, but generally radiography is used to identify changes to bone structure.

Radiographs are used to diagnose pathological changes occurring in the foot, in combination with a full clinical examination, and sometimes in conjunction with other diagnostic procedures. They can be used to assess the progress, severity and likely prognosis (outcome) of a condition, and in some cases they will be used to rule out certain conditions.

From the changes seen, radiographs may give an indication of the duration of a condition. For instance, some bone fractures may not be visible initially, either due to lack of displacement or to the alignment of the x-ray beam, and they only become evident when new bone has been laid down in the repair process.

Radiographs can also be used to assess hoof balance and the relationship of the internal structures to this, which can provide information to the farrier for specific trimming or shoeing protocols.

Some people use radiographs as part of the pre-purchase examination of a horse, but because there are frequently different opinions on what they show, this can be problematic.

Radiographic Views

The name of a radiographic view refers to the direction of the x-ray beam, from the x-ray machine to the film cassette. The positional terms can be long and technical, so the names of the views are usually abbreviated or given a simpler title. The direction is very often controlled by practical considerations for the safety of the horse, the operators and the expensive x-ray equipment. Because the result

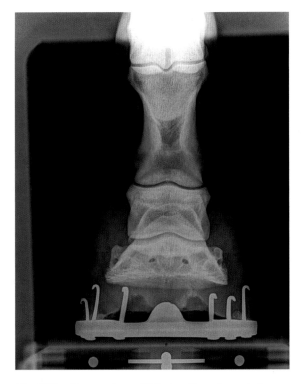

Fig. 185 Dorsopalmar (DP) standing view – taken from directly in front of the foot with the cassette placed vertically against the back of the fetlock (still sometimes referred to as 'anteroposterior' or 'AP'). Particularly useful for assessing mediolateral balance.

is two-dimensional, a very similar image is obtained if the beam is in the directly opposite direction.

The lateromedial (LM) view (commonly referred to just as the 'lateral' view) of the foot is the commonest radiograph taken of the horse (*see* Fig. 184): it is taken directly from the side with the cassette placed next to the inside of the leg. Because the x-ray film is contained inside a cassette, the bottom of the foot will be missed unless the foot is raised up on a block.

To obtain diagnostic radiographs, correct positioning of the x-ray equipment in relation to what is being studied in the foot is necessary. A single radiograph is often difficult to interpret

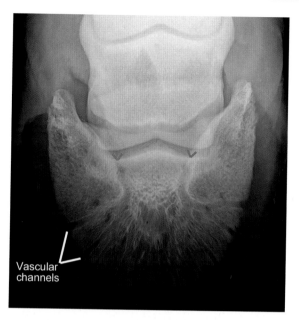

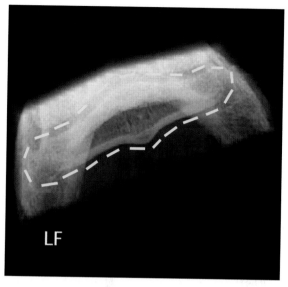

Fig. 188   The navicular bone (and the palmar processes of P3) can be imaged with a 'skyline' view (palmaroproximal-palmarodistal view): the horse's foot is placed on a cassette and the x-ray beam is aimed downwards behind the pastern. (Image courtesy Liphook Vet Hospital)

Fig. 186   Dorsopalmar upright pedal view (dorsoproximal-palmarodistal oblique): this view is taken with the x-ray beam horizontal and the fetlock and foot flexed so that the bottom of the foot rests against a vertically placed cassette. It is used to look for changes to the structure of P3. (The arrow-heads indicate where the palmar digital arteries enter P3. These two arteries join together in the 'terminal arch' inside the bone and smaller arteries radiate out from this, passing through vascular channels to then anastomose and form the circumflex artery of the sole, to supply blood to the laminae and the sole.)

because it is just a two-dimensional image, which is why multiple views are usually taken. Sometimes additional radiographs will be taken from different angles to those described above (oblique views), to highlight a particular area of concern.

Radiographic Interpretation

I suggested to a farrier that if eight vets examined a radiograph there would probably be eight different diagnoses. 'Ten,' was his reply, 'because two will have changed their

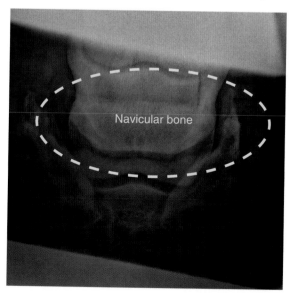

Fig. 187   To image the navicular bone, the foot is positioned at a slightly different angle to the dorsopalmar upright view, and a higher exposure is used. The edge of the navicular bone can be made out within the dotted area.

mind before the end!' In the clinical situation, when symptoms can be correlated with possible changes seen on the radiographs, this would not usually be the case, but including the 'joke' seemed to be a good way to indicate how difficult interpreting radiographs can be.

It takes experience to work out how the shape of bones and the way they overlap affects the way they appear on the radiograph, and also how different positioning of the foot can alter this. You will find that the more radiographs you look at, the better you will become at identifying differences, so start by studying the few examples I have included, and if you are interested, there are plenty of examples on the internet that you can study.

The Use of Radio-opaque Materials

Metal objects have commonly been used to mark the foot so that specific points can be identified on the radiograph, but because modern digital images can be manipulated on the computer, thus making it easier to identify these points, many vets no longer apply markers. In many cases this is adequate, but there are situations where markers are undoubtedly of benefit, the most obvious of these being in cases of laminitis, where metal markers or barium paste undoubtedly make

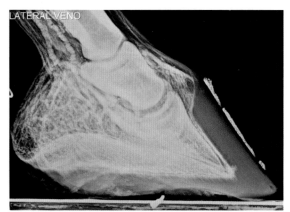

Fig. 189 *Venogram: when an iodine-based liquid is injected into a vein, the venous system can be seen on a radiograph. (Image courtesy Dr Amy Rucker)*

interpretation of the changes much easier. An advantage of modern digital x-ray equipment is the inclusion of software, for example the Metron System, to help measure features on the radiograph, and using external markers will improve the accuracy of any measurements made involving the hoof wall.

Barium paste is suitable for external marking of the foot, but iodine-based liquids are needed for studying the blood supply or investigating soft tissue injuries of the foot – for example to try to determine the depth and direction of a nail penetration into the sole or frog. Both of these liquids are radio-opaque, with the elements iodine and barium having the ability to absorb the energy of x-rays, thus showing up as white on a radiograph.

Arteriograms are obtained by taking radiographs after contrast medium has been injected into an artery, but are rarely used to study the arterial supply of the equine foot; however, the injection of contrast medium into a vein to produce a venogram is becoming more popular, particularly when dealing with cases of laminitis. The procedure is not particularly complicated, but both the technique and the timing of the radiographs after injection of the radio-opaque liquid have to be very precise. Because the venous plexuses of the foot are distributed so they are easily compressed (to help return blood to the heart), changes in the position of the foot will affect the distribution of blood (and the radio-opaque liquid) in the foot – which is one reason why interpreting the venogram is challenging.

FURTHER INVESTIGATIVE PROCEDURES

Scintigraphy (Radio-isotope scintigraphy)

When radio-isotopes (radioactive substances that emit gamma irradiation) are injected

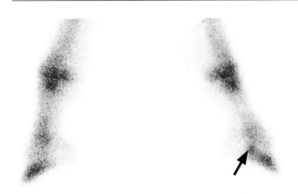

Fig. 190 Scintigraphy – the difference between the left and right image (left and right foot) is increased uptake (a 'hot spot') in the navicular bone of the right fore (arrow). (Courtesy Jane Boswell)

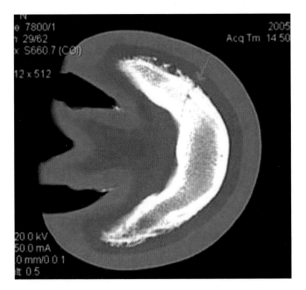

Fig. 191 Each CT image shows a 'slice' through a structure. This CT image identifies a fracture to P3 (arrow). By combining CT images, a three-dimensional image of the structure can be produced. (Image courtesy Dr Roger Smith)

intravenously, they are taken up by the tissues and their distribution in the body can be monitored by measuring radiation using a 'gamma camera'. Emissions picked up immediately following the injection identify soft tissue uptake, and then those picked up

at a later stage identify uptake by the bones. The result is a two-dimensional image that shows 'hot spots' where there has been greater uptake of the radio-active material, indicating an area of inflammation or repair, and if this is in the bone, may be followed up with further radiography, CT or MRI (*see* below).

X-ray Computed Tomography (CT scan)

This uses x-rays to produce a three-dimensional image. The x-ray source and the receptor plate are contained in a ring-like structure that allows them to rotate around the part of the body placed in the middle of the ring. Multiple radiographic images are taken, and the computer then converts all these two-dimensional images into a three-dimensional one. A general anaesthetic is required for this procedure when used for horses, since the patient needs to remain completely still.

Magnetic Resonance Imaging (MRI)

I don't believe there is any simple way of explaining magnetic resonance imaging, but in brief, 'resonance' is energy produced in the cells of the body when they are subjected to a strong magnetic field and radio frequency waves, and an MRI scanner is able to measure the energy generated by the different tissues and convert this to an image. By altering the strength and frequency of the electromagnetic field the operator is able to manipulate the parameters on the scanner to produce images that display a contrast between different tissues and can identify pathological changes. The two basic types of scan are referred to as T1- and T2-weighted, differentiating between fat and water on the image, with fat appearing as light, and water as dark in the T1-weighted scan, and the opposite of this for T2.

When MRI was used in horses initially, the

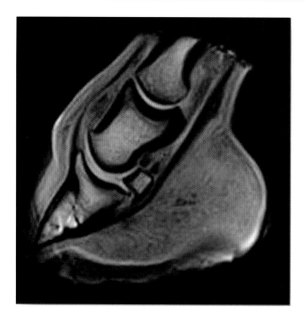

Fig. 192   A T1-weighted MRI sagittal scan of a 'normal' horse's foot performed under standing sedation using a low field (0.27 Tesla) magnet. (Courtesy Jane Boswell)

equipment available meant that it could only be carried out with the horse under general anaesthetic, but equipment is now available to image the lower limb in the standing sedated horse, which reduces the cost – though it is still an expensive procedure.

Infrared Thermography (or Thermal Imaging, Medical Thermology)

Thermography is a technique using a thermal imaging camera to detect infra-red radiation emitted from the surface of an object. The camera amplifies and then processes the signal to convert it into a visible image which can be seen on a screen or downloaded to produce a 'thermogram'. These show up as different colours on the image for different levels of emission, indicating which areas are

hotter or colder. Comparison of the different temperatures in the feet may be useful, but for an individual foot there are physiological as well as environmental reasons for changes in its temperature, which makes it difficult to identify actual pathological problems. In experienced hands it may be able to locate specific problems, but in many cases it will provide little more information than a thorough clinical examination.

Ultrasound Scan (Ultrasound Imaging or Medical Ultrasonography)

The simple explanation of ultrasound imaging is that sound waves are directed at the part of the body being investigated, and then the 'echo' from the tissues is recorded, and converted to produce an image that can be seen on a screen (like the baby scans that ladies have during pregnancy).

Although widely available, these sound waves cannot penetrate the hoof wall and have limited penetration of the frog, so the use of ultrasonography for diagnosing problems in horses' feet is limited. Scanning from behind the pastern down between the heel bulbs or through the frog from the underside of the foot may identify problems in the navicular bursa or in the DDFT. One area where it can be useful is in identifying damage in the collateral ligaments of the coffin joint (*see* Figs 15 and 19).

Arthroscopy: Endoscopy of Joints

It is possible to examine inside the coffin joint and the navicular bursa with an arthroscope. Using fibre-optics, light can be shone into the joint or bursa, and the internal structures can be seen directly through the eyepiece, or shown on a video screen. The arthroscope is introduced into the joint and allows investigation of these

Table 1: Investigative Procedures

Modality	Use	Availability	Cost	Safety	GA	Tissues	Specificity
Nerve block	Locate	+++	+			All	++
Joint block	Locate	+++	+			Joint	++
Radiography	Diagnosis	+++	+	Radiation		Bone (+ soft)	++
Scintigraphy **	Locate	+	++	Radiation		Bone (+ soft)	++
CT scan **	Diagnosis	+	+++	Radiation	+	Bone (+ soft)	+++
MRI **	Diagnosis	+	+++		+/-	Bone (+ soft)	+++
Thermography	Locate	+	+				+
Ultrasonography	Diagnosis	++	+			Ligament/tendon	++
Arthroscopy **	Diagnosis	+	+++		+	Joints + bursa	+++

Table 1 'Use' – Some methods generally need further investigations before a specific diagnosis can be made, and these are identified with 'locate' rather than 'diagnosis'.

GA = general anaesthetic

*** = restricted to use in a veterinary hospital*

cavities, and via a second entry point, facilitates the surgical removal of damaged cartilage and flushing of the joint. A general anaesthetic is required to carry out arthroscopy and arthroscopic surgery of the coffin joint in the horse.

Table 1 provides a list of the methods used to investigate lameness problems in horses. In most cases, the first line of investigation will involve nerve and/or joint blocks and radiography. Beyond this, what procedures are used will depend on a number of factors:

- Whether it can only be used in a hospital or if it is available 'out in the field'
- The availability of the equipment
- Whether a bone or soft tissue injury is suspected
- If a general anaesthetic is required, where the risk factor as well as the cost needs to be considered

- The comparative cost-effectiveness of the equipment available
- The safety of the procedure for horse, handlers and equipment
- The cost of the procedure

All these modalities require experience, not only in how to use them, but also in being able to interpret the information they provide, to identify what is normal as well as what is abnormal.

RADIOGRAPHY IN THE LAMINITIS CASE

Radiography is used in laminitis cases to ascertain the extent of any changes that have occurred, to provide information that can be used in the management of the affected feet, and for monitoring the progress (and prognosis) of the condition. In cases of laminitis, alteration in the relationship of P3 to all the other foot structures is equally as important as any changes seen in the bone. By altering the radiographic exposure, some of these other structures can be identified on radiographs (*see* Fig. 193).

The first thing a vet is likely to comment on, from a foot radiograph of a horse with laminitis, is 'degrees of rotation' of P3, but it is not always clear what the vet is referring to: rotation of P3 in relation to what? (*See* Fig. 194) 'Rotation of P3' is most commonly used to refer to the difference in angle between the deviated hoof

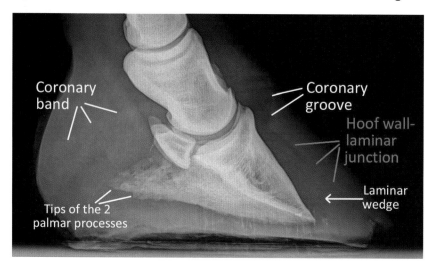

Fig. 193 By changing the contrast and definition of a radiograph, different foot structures can be identified. In this radiograph, the junction between the dorsal hoof wall (lighter) and the underlying soft tissues (darker), including the line of the coronary groove, is evident, as well as the faint line of the coronary band from the change in density between hoof and skin.

Fig. 194 'Rotation of P3' is generally used to describe the difference in angle between the deviated hoof wall 'e' and the dorsal surface of P3 'b', but sometimes it is used for the difference in angle between the line of the pastern bones 'a' and the dorsal surface of P3 'b', when the angle of the P3 is steeper than the pastern angle. Some vets refer to any increase in the palmar angle (the angle between the solar border of P3 'c' and the ground 'g') as 'rotation'.

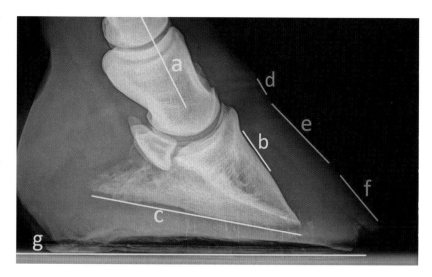

The degree of capsular rotation is likely to be the most relevant but will depend on which part of the wall the angle of rotation is measured from – 'd', 'e' or 'f'. Because this is a digital radiograph, the operator will have been able to alter the definition of the image to help identify the outer surface of the dorsal wall, but it is easier to do, and more accurate, if the dorsal wall is 'marked', either with a line of barium paste or a flexible metal wire ('d' is the estimated line of the new growth of the dorsal wall, 'e' the line of the separated wall, and 'f' the distal wall, which has been rasped by the farrier).

Fig. 195 The hoof-lamellar zone (HL) is the distance between the outer surface of the dorsal wall and the surface of P3. Generally the HL distance is given as two numbers, measurements taken at the upper and lower parts of the dorsal surface of P3. There can be a significant difference between the two measurements when there is (capsular) rotation of P3.

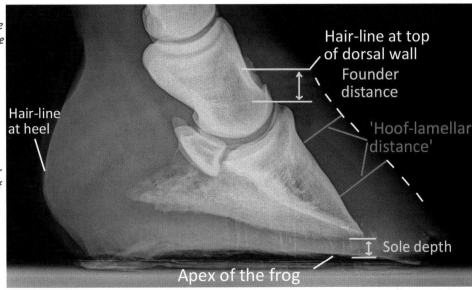

To measure the 'founder distance' accurately requires a dorsal wall marker to extend to the very top of the dorsal wall (estimated on this radiograph).

The sole depth is the distance between the tip of P3 and the bottom of the sole (this can be made clearer if marked with barium paste), and includes the width of the solar corium as well as the thickness of the horny sole. If there is still some concavity of the sole, a dark area (air) is visible between the sole and block of wood the foot is on (see above) or shoe, if shod. If the sole has 'dropped' there will be no air space visible in the unshod foot, and if shod, may appear to be even thinner if the sole has become convex and the sole surface is hidden by the shoe.

wall and the dorsal surface of P3, sometimes referred to as 'capsular rotation', but some vets refer to the degrees of difference between the line of the pastern bones and the dorsal surface of P3, when the angle of the P3 is steeper than the pastern angle, sometimes referred to as 'phalangeal rotation'. To confuse things further, some vets refer to any increase in the palmar angle as 'degrees of rotation'.

The palmar angle will increase when there is accelerated heel growth or if less heel is removed at trimming. Phalangeal rotation will depend on the heel height (increasing the dorsal angle of P3), but is also affected by the position of the limb when the radiograph is taken, which will produce a different pastern angle (phalangeal rotation is generally only used when the angle of P3 is greater than the pastern angle – *see* Figs 5

and 202). The degree of capsular rotation is likely to be the most relevant description of bone displacement, but this will depend on which part of the wall the angle of rotation is measured from (*see* Fig. 194). Vets need to make it clear (or the owner should ask) what they are referring to when talking about 'degrees of rotation'.

Other features are regularly measured on radiographs of feet with chronic laminitis, to identify the extent of the separation and the displacement of P3, which can be used to compare with later radiographs as laminitis progresses and may be used to indicate the likely prognosis of the case.

In acute laminitis, the first measurable changes on radiographs will be an increase in the hoof-lamellar (HL) zone, as the laminae start to separate. The HL distance is the distance between the outer surface of the dorsal wall and the surface of P3. This includes the thickness of the hoof and the vascular sensitive laminae, and any laminar wedge material, when present (*see* Fig. 195).

The 'founder distance' is sometimes used to refer to the vertical distance between the top of the dorsal wall and the top of the extensor process of P3, and indicates the extent of displacement (sinking) of P3 relative to the hoof capsule. A founder distance of over 15mm (normally <10mm) has been reported to be a poor prognostic indicator in cases of laminitis.

The distance between the tip of P3 and the ground is of significance in laminitis cases.

This distance includes the depth of the sole providing protection to the tip of P3, and the ground clearance between the sole and the ground, a measure of whether the sole has dropped relative to the hoof. Normally the sole thickness is around 15mm.

Identifying the apex of the frog by applying some form of marker (a drawing pin is often used) will help with correct placement of a shoe, which is particularly important when applying a heart-bar shoe.

Being able to identify the hair-line at the bulb of the heel by applying a marker can also provide some useful information (*see* The PAD, Chapter 12).

11 Internal Foot Problems

Although some of the conditions described in this chapter may be diagnosed from the symptoms exhibited by the horse, because they are occurring inside the hoof structure, many of them will require the investigatory procedures described in Chapter 10 in order to make the diagnosis.

FOREIGN BODY PENETRATION

Fortunately it is rare for a foreign body to penetrate the sole or frog deep enough as to involve P3, the DDFT or the navicular bursa, but those that do can become life-threatening for the horse. Infection of these important structures deep inside the foot are very difficult to treat, and even with a general anaesthetic and debridement and flushing, some horses will remain permanently crippled. The earlier these are operated on, the better the chance of a good outcome, and the more knowledge of the direction and depth of the penetration of a foreign body, the greater the likelihood that a vet will be able to make that early referral.

Occasionally a foreign object is found embedded in the sole or frog, and the immediate reaction is to remove it as quickly as

possible – but it is important to stay calm and to leave it in place until the full situation has been considered:

- What is the nature of the foreign body? Is it a nail, a piece of wood or a large flint? Can the likely depth of penetration be assessed from the size and shape of the object?
- What part of the foot is the foreign body embedded in? Is it in the middle third of the foot where it could penetrate the deep flexor tendon or the navicular bursa, or in front of the frog where it might damage the bone?
- How lame is the horse and how distressed is it ? A horse is likely to be reluctant to put its foot down if the foreign body has penetrated

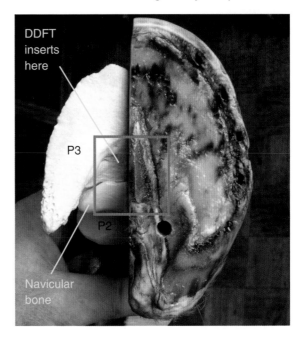

DDFT inserts here

P3

P2

Navicular bone

Fig. 196 The danger of complications following foreign body penetration is greatest in the red boxed area. A sharp object penetrating through the DDFT into the coffin joint or navicular bursa can be particularly difficult to deal with.

the dermis or deeper, so only if it is very slightly lame can we surmise that there is only a superficial penetration.

- What are the chances that the foreign body will penetrate further if the horse stays where it is, and a vet can be contacted to attend urgently?
- If you are alone and have no means of contacting anyone to help, what are the chances of the foreign body penetrating deeper if the horse is to be walked at all?

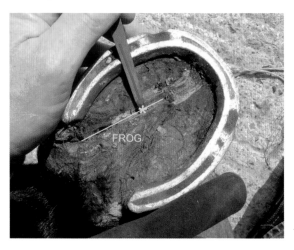

Fig. 197   This pony had a nail removed from this site: it was referred to a hospital and operated on that night when radiographs revealed that the navicular bursa had been penetrated. (The pony recovered fully from this.)

Only having considered all these things should a decision be made as to whether to remove the foreign body or not. If the decision is made to remove it, carefully note the position and direction of the penetration, and if you have a camera (or a mobile phone), take a photograph prior to removal. Examine the foreign body for any blood since this could give an indication of the depth of penetration.

Where the situation allows, the penetration hole should be flushed with clean water or a mild antiseptic after the foreign body is removed, and the foot bandaged to prevent any dirt getting up the hole. Small hole

punctures, particularly those involving the frog, will close over rapidly, and it is likely that flushing will only be possible immediately following removal of the foreign body.

If not referred for further investigation and surgery, treatment is likely to include analgesics, antibiotics and protection for tetanus, if the horse has not previously been vaccinated.

FOOT ABSCESSES

Deep Abscesses

The hoof, sole and frog provide a significant barrier to penetration, but when infection does

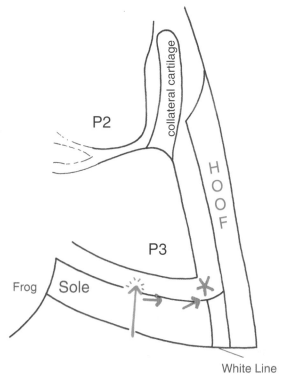

Fig. 198   Cut to show the side of the foot (similar to Fig. 120). Penetration through the sole to cause an abscess. Pus tends to push between the sole layers, towards the outer wall, and will most commonly channel around the perimeter of the foot (see red star '') see Fig. 200.*

Fig. 199   An abscess occurring after dirt and infection gain entry through a damaged white line generally spreads around the perimeter of the sole, but it may spread up between the laminae to break out at the coronary band, particularly when the defect also involves a crack in the wall.

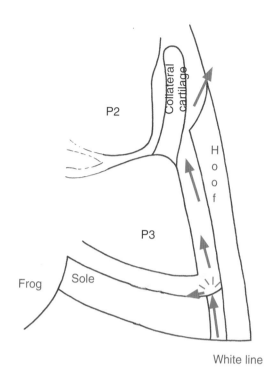

gain entry, pus cannot easily escape and an abscess will develop in the sensitive underlying dermis. In most cases, foreign bodies that puncture the sole and frog will only reach as far as the sensitive dermis, sometimes because of the size and shape of the object, but also because of evasive action taken by the horse in response to the pain. Sometimes it will go lame immediately due to the traumatic damage to the dermis and then deteriorate as an abscess forms, but at other times it may be two or three days before pus builds up and lameness becomes obvious.

Because of the inflammation, and pus that is accumulating inside the relatively rigid structure of the hoof, these abscesses can be extremely painful and the horse is likely to exhibit the more obvious diagnostic symptoms: a strong digital pulse, a hot foot, altered foot placement and possibly some leg oedema. With no means of escape for the pus, the pain persists until an opening is made to release it, or it finds a place to burst out.

Superficial Abscesses

Superficial abscesses occur where there is separation at the dermal-epidermal junction. Infection can reach the sensitive dermis through damaged or diseased horn structures, most commonly via defects in the 'white line'. Dirt pushing up through a split or defect in the 'white line' causes an inflammatory response when it reaches the dermis, and the pus formed is unable to escape because of the dirt that has

built up behind it. For some of these superficial abscesses, it seems that it is the dirt continually being pushed up into the defect that is more of a problem than any infection introduced.

Dirt and infection may also gain entry through cracks in the bottom of the hoof wall or from superficial damage to the sole or frog, and this type of abscess can also result from a misplaced shoe nail.

These abscesses can still be very painful, but as a rule are a lot less so than deeper ones, and if a horse with this type of abscess is stabled and rested the lameness may well settle down, which is a pattern of lameness that does not suggest an abscess. However, when these cases are turned out again, more dirt pushing up through the defect causes the lameness to return. As the dirt and pus spreads, it uses the weak attachment between the layers of sole as a means of escape, rather than the junction of the dermis and epidermis. This still causes pain, due to pressure on the underlying dermal layer, but not as much as when the dermis is directly involved.

These cases may have a change in strength of the digital pulse, but it is usually less obvious than with deeper abscesses, and in some cases may not be noticeable.

Symptoms of a Foot Abscess

Lameness may be the only symptom to see, and the pattern and severity of the lameness will depend on the stage of abscess formation, the type and site of the infection, and the individual horse's tolerance to pain. For this reason there is a very wide variation in how a foot abscess manifests itself. However, there are some features that can make them easier to identify than many other foot problems.

- A foot abscess will cause a 'weight-bearing' lameness, accompanied by the horse lifting its head as it puts weight on the foot.
- A horse may alter its stance, foot placement or stride length, to reduce pressure on the abscess. If the toe is painful, the horse is likely to take a lengthened stride but pick the foot up earlier to avoid putting weight on the toe. If the pain is in the back of the (palmar) foot, the horse will try to avoid weighting the heel, and will have a shortened forward stride; more painful than this and it will walk only on the toe.
- A persistently warm hoof as compared to the other three is likely to indicate inflammation occurring somewhere in the foot; however, it is not specific for an abscess.
- There will generally be a palpable increase in the strength of the digital pulse. A strong digital pulse is also regularly found with laminitis, but in most cases this is present in more than one limb, which helps to differentiate it. The problem occurs when laminitis affects only one foot, and this can cause it to be misdiagnosed as an abscess.

To examine the foot properly, it needs to be thoroughly cleaned. If the horse is shod, the shoe will cover up any defects in the white line, which is a common site of entry for infection, but a crack at the bottom of the hoof, or a split in the sole or frog may be found, indicating where infection could have gained entry.

Withdrawal of the foot when pressure is applied over a visible defect will help to confirm if this is the site of the problem. Thumb pressure may be sufficient for this, but careful use of hoof-testers may be needed to locate the painful area.

If the horse has been recently shod, an abscess may have developed due to nail penetration into the sensitive part of the foot when the shoe was fitted. Check the position of the nails.

The coronary band should be closely checked and palpated to see if there is a painful spot where an abscess is about to burst, or a damp horizontal split where it already has. Occasionally there is swelling of the coronet and pastern, and this may extend further up the leg on the side of the abscess. This is oedema fluid, which may be identified by the indentation left in the swollen area after it has been squeezed and released. This will collect partly because of the extra fluid drawn into the inflamed area around an abscess, but also because less fluid is dispersed as a result of the reduced mechanical pumping when the horse does not weight the painful foot in the normal way.

Having ascertained that a lame horse with a hot foot and a pronounced digital pulse is likely to have an abscess, working out exactly where it is and what has caused it usually ends up being the task of a vet and/or farrier.

Progression of Abscesses

Deep abscesses will continue to be painful until the pus finds an escape route. Infection that gains entry through skin is localized by a fibrous wall that is produced to protect the surrounding tissue; the pus is eventually released at the skin surface once this abscess has thinned and burst.

While in most cases the foot appears able to localize an infection, finding a means of escape for the pus is potentially more of a problem. With the entry wound closed over or plugged with dirt, the easiest route of escape for the pus is by forcing its way between the layers of formed sole closest to the dermis. There may be some local spread under the sole close to the abscess, but in most cases pus pushes its way to the perimeter of the sole, where it works its way around the foot till it reaches the heel. The shape of the heel angle provides the easiest escape route and the pus bursts out at the bulb of the heel.

Fig. 200   Left: the red arrow shows where the sole was penetrated, and the blue arrow where the abscess burst (with evidence of discharge down the wall). Right: eight days later, and the extent of the abscess tract is exposed (see the broken red line). The blue 'X' shows where the pus spread up between the laminae to burst out at the heel.

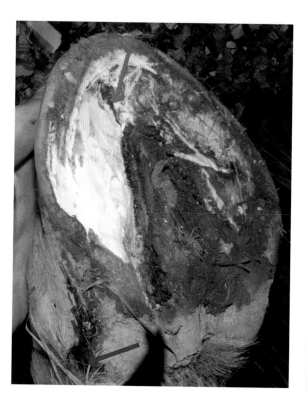

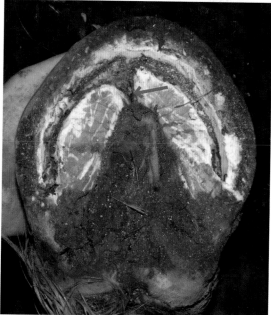

Abscesses resulting from hoof cracks that reach the laminae may escape directly up the wall, to burst out at the coronet above the split. Certain types of infection can also spread up the wall – for example, pseudomonas can activate local enzymes, thereby allowing the infection to move up between the laminae very rapidly. Those that spread up the wall are generally extremely painful, putting pressure on the laminae beside the tract, and particularly so as pus forces its way through the skin/ hoof junction at the coronary band. When the abscess bursts there is a brief break in hoof growth which results in a horizontal crack; this will move down with the wall as new hoof grows down connected above it.

Abscesses underneath the frog, if unable to escape locally, will invariably spread towards the back of the foot and burst out at the base of the frog.

With deep abscesses, once the pus has found an escape route, the injured dermis is generally able to heal and the tract moves away from the sensitive dermis as new sole is produced. With superficial sub-solar abscesses, it is possible

for them to settle down, with new sole being produced to isolate the abscess, which then 'grows out' with the sole; more commonly, however, mud and dirt keep pushing up through the defect and the abscess continues to be a problem, eventually requiring investigation and attention.

Abscesses and Laminitis

'Laminitic Abscess' Following Acute Laminitis

'Abscesses' that follow acute laminitis are different from those discussed above, because they are not the result of infection but develop in the space created when the laminae separate. (Pus formation is not necessarily a response to infection, and the build-up of fluid and the collection of large numbers of white cells to get rid of dead and damaged tissue is still referred to as 'pus'.)

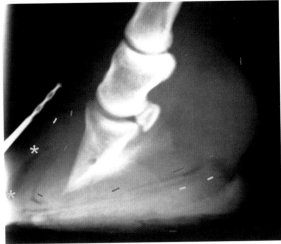

Fig. 202   There are two dark lines where separation has occurred in two serious laminitis episodes. These lines (below the red marks and above the yellow marks) extend down the wall and underneath P3. Between the yellow stars is a cavity – a laminitis 'abscess' that may have burst out at the coronary band or the heel, since the separation extends from the surface of the dorsal wall right to the heel.

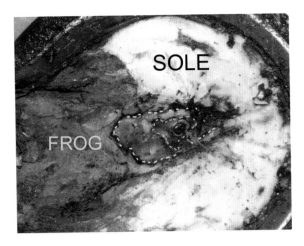

Fig. 201   Infection from a puncture wound (red arrow) near the point of the frog has caused separation of several layers (broken orange and yellow lines), at different stages of the process. Pus was able to escape locally, which is why spread between the layers was limited.

The different explanations put forward as to how these abscesses form come from the different opinions on the pathophysiology of the laminitis process. Some believe that inflammation causes the laminae to separate because of pressure build-up of the inflammatory fluid in the dermis, but I believe it is more likely that the 'abscess' forms after the laminae have separated and are then mechanically pulled apart, after which inflammatory fluid fills the space. In more severe cases of laminitis, when there has been complete separation of the laminae, this fluid-filled space may be evident as an obvious dark line between the hoof and the bone on radiographs. This is usually just referred to as 'separation', and only when it bursts out at the coronet or the heel does it seem to be called an 'abscess'.

In most cases the foot can deal with the fluid that fills the cavity without having to release it, unlike infected abscesses, and although when it bursts out some suggest 'it is the body's way of getting rid of the necrotic (dead) tissue', it may be more to do with changes in pressure distribution, since some of them seem to break out shortly after a foot has been trimmed. 'Bursting out' is most likely in feet with greater separation, occurring at the coronary band when displacement of P3 has caused it to distort sufficiently to prevent new horn to grow down attached to the laminae; however, at other times the abscess may open up at the heel.

Abscesses in Chronic Laminitis

Change to the 'white line' produced by distorted terminal papillae following laminitis makes these feet prone to abscessation. The 'white line' ends up being wider and weaker than in normal feet, and splits in it are common. Dirt and infection can gain entry through these defects to produce the superficial abscesses described above. Management of abscesses in

these feet is not quite so easy due to laminar wedge material up the wall, and may be further complicated by new episodes of laminitis, so treatment must always include suitable management to control IR and laminitis as well as for any current abscess.

Dealing with Laminitic Abscesses

Acute laminitis 'abscesses' are characterized by large areas of separation of the epidermis (laminae) rather than the localized area that occurs with other abscesses, and in this situation, opening them up could expose an extensive area of sensitive dermis. It could allow the entry of dirt and infection to already compromised tissue, and particularly for the sole, exposed dermis will be liable to physical damage.

Six to eight weeks after a laminitic attack, the farrier may encounter not just bruising but a cavity in the sole. These are areas of sole separation that occurred at the time of the laminitis attack, and provided the horse has 'recovered' from the laminitis episode, can generally be opened up safely at that stage, because new sole has formed underneath to provide protection.

Abscesses occurring in chronic laminitis, when not associated with a further acute episode, are dealt with as other infected abscesses.

Dorsal Wall Resection

Some vets cut away a section of the dorsal wall as part of their treatment for laminitis. This is done to take pressure off the coronary band to try to allow new wall to grow down attached. Generally a large section of dorsal wall is removed, leaving a strip of hoof at the coronary band; however, some vets now remove a strip at the top while leaving the lower wall to provide stability.

A resection of the distal wall is generally carried out beyond six weeks after an acute laminitis attack, when there is sufficient overall stability to the foot, because if the side walls break down, a dorsal wall resection can end in disaster. To avoid this, it is necessary to provide additional support, which traditionally (over the past thirty years) has been with the application of a heart-bar shoe, but can also be achieved with a hoof cast. A dorsal wall resection is also used in the treatment of seedy toe and the surgical removal of keratomas.

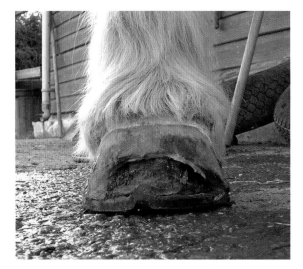

Fig. 203   The separated dorsal wall has been removed (dorsal wall resection), at a stage, in this foot, when the dermis is already protected by a layer of keratinized tissue that has subsequently dried and hardened. (Left fore foot of a Welsh Cob.)

Recurrent Abscesses

There are several possible reasons why an abscess recurs. If this is after only a short time, it is most likely because the abscess hasn't resolved and the drainage hole has become blocked, or because more dirt has pushed up through the hole to cause further separation.

In laminitis cases, recurrent abscesses occur either because the laminitis recurs, or infections gain access intermittently through the damaged 'white line'.

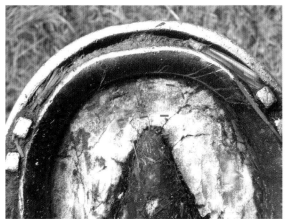

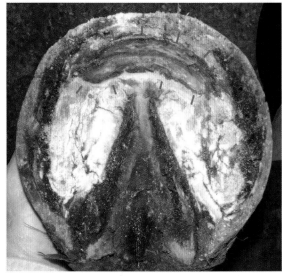

Fig. 204   Top: lame six weeks after a laminitis attack. The sole at the toe was thinned to release fluid (possibly not suitable at this stage if in a wet environment.) Below: four weeks later and the full cavity is exposed with healthy sole underneath.

Infection in P3 can cause recurrent abscesses. This may occur directly from a foreign body, or in cases of laminitis, when the tip of P3 becomes infected following 'penetration' of the sole. Rarely, a penetrating foreign body such as a blackthorn or a small piece of flint remains embedded in the dermis, and an abscess can recur until this is located and removed. These can be difficult to identify since the foreign object will generally not show up on radiographs.

Management and Treatment of Abscesses

Very often the vet will attend the lame horse before an abscess has burst and will provide a means of escape for the pus. Just providing an opening for drainage may be all that is done on the first visit, particularly if the foot is very painful. At a later time it may be suitable to remove the separated sole and expose any escape tract, to allow these to harden.

Abscesses that travel up the wall are more of a problem to deal with since it is often difficult to open up the defect sufficiently, and searching up the wall puts pressure on the adjoining laminae, which the horse strongly resents.

The advantages of opening an abscess are as follows.

- It allows the pus to escape and rapidly gives pain relief to the horse.
- The healing process can be speeded up, avoiding the necessity of, and the damage caused by, the formation of the escape tracts.
- With protection, the horse is likely to get back to work much more quickly.

However, there are also disadvantages. Nature does not provide an escape route on the ground surface of the foot because this would quickly become blocked by dirt, and this is a potential problem if an abscess is opened on the bottom of the foot. Also, when the newly formed sole layers are exposed they will initially be sensitive, so the foot will require some form of protective covering applied to it, and in some cases this may be necessary for some time.

If damaged dermis is exposed, it may protrude through the hole that has been made in the sole, and as well as this fleshy material

being more prone to direct damage, it may be 'pinched' by the rigid sole around the hole, which is painful. Thinning of the rim of any hole made in the sole, to make it more flexible, can help to avoid this.

These disadvantages can be overcome by covering and protecting any holes in the sole to prevent them becoming blocked, and this can also allow exposed sole layers to harden and become less sensitive. Protection by bandaging or by putting a boot on the foot needs to be continued until things have resolved. At this stage, if the horse is normally shod, a pad can be fitted under a shoe to give added protection to any thinned areas of sole.

It is important that any abscess occurring as a consequence of laminitis, whether acute or chronic, has suitable changes in management to control it.

The Use of Poultices and Bandages

Sometimes it is not possible to locate an abscess, and nature must take its course, with the pus having to find its own means of escape; applying a poultice to the foot may help it to do so. A poultice provides a means of applying heat to a foot to try to 'draw' an abscess, encouraging it to burst. Commercially prepared poultices are now available, but in the past, heated kaolin or bran wrapped over the foot would often be used to apply heat. Even if the poultice does not speed up the natural process and cause the abscess to burst, it will soften the horn structures and this may make it easier for the vet to locate it and provide an escape route for the pus.

Once an abscess has been opened up, repeated application of wet poultices is unlikely to be of benefit, and particularly if left on constantly, will keep the horn tissues soft, which is not desirable. Wetness will keep thinned soles sensitive, and laminitis cases that have the tip of P3 resting on the sole are generally more comfortable when the sole is allowed to harden.

Once an abscess tract has been opened up to allow drainage, after an initial wet poultice or foot soaking to help clean out the affected area, it is usually better to use a dry dressing to keep mud and dirt from penetrating or blocking up any opening, and to allow the horn structures to harden.

Cotton wool (absorbent cotton) is excellent for allowing pus to soak away while preventing dirt getting in, and I would recommend plugging holes with this, under any dressing, in case a bandage or boot comes off. Once opened up and the pus released, most horses will benefit from movement, so can be turned out as soon as they are comfortable and provided the foot is suitably protected. However, for those laminitic abscesses that are the result of an acute episode, confinement must be continued until P3 has been stabilized. Most horses will show considerable improvement in lameness within twenty-four to forty-eight hours of an abscess being opened up. If a horse continues to be severely lame, the case should be reassessed and the diagnosis re-evaluated, which may involve further investigation.

Medication

Tetanus antitoxin: Should be given if a horse with a foot abscess has not previously been vaccinated against tetanus. (Tetanus is caused by the toxin of the anaerobic bacteria *Clostridium tetani*.)

Analgesics: Should be given to relieve the pain caused by an abscess. The release of pus, either by opening up the abscess or once an abscess has burst, will rapidly reduce the pain and the analgesic dose can usually be quickly reduced or stopped.

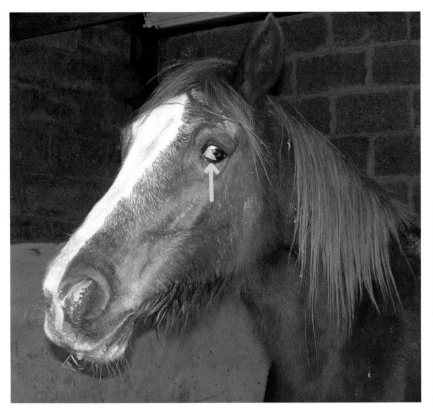

Fig. 205 This horse developed tetanus, through infection of an unseen wound under its jaw. When a horse with tetanus is stimulated, many muscles of the body go into spasm, including the muscle of the 'third eyelid'. 'Lockjaw' is a name used for tetanus in man, because the muscles of the jaw go into spasm. This horse was unable to eat or drink.

Antibiotics: The use of antibiotics to treat any abscess before it has burst is controversial, particularly in diseases that produce abscesses in other parts of the body, such as strangles (caused by Strep. equi) and Dryland distemper/ pigeon fever (caused by *C. Pseudotuberculosis*). Although commonly used antibiotics are able to kill the bacteria involved in these diseases, they are unable to reach them in the centre of an abscess, and treating an abscess with antibiotics can just delay the resolution of the problem. For foot abscesses, even if an antibiotic is able to reach the infection, the ones in common use are unlikely to be able to kill the type of bacteria (anaerobic) that are present.

In many cases antibiotics will therefore be of limited benefit. They are most likely to help if they are given at the time of a sole penetration, or when an abscess has been opened and damaged dermis is exposed, when the antibiotic will at least reach the damaged tissue. They should also be used in cases where an unopened abscess is making the horse toxic.

Antibiotics will be of no benefit for superficial abscesses, where what is required is exposure of the abscess tract and the prevention of any more dirt getting in.

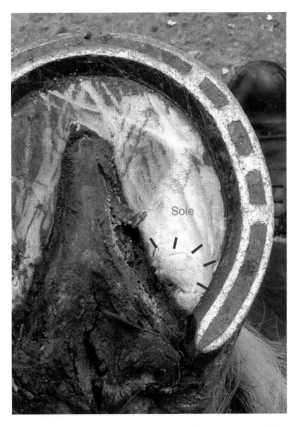

Fig. 206   A keratoma in the bar. This was successfully removed under general anaesthetic. The left fore of a Welsh Cob.

KERATOMA

Keratomas are made up of abnormal keratinized tissue and are found on the inside of the hoof wall, most commonly as a tubular strip extending from the coronary band down to the sole. They are not tumours, although they are commonly referred to as such, but are thought to be formed from an abnormal, localized response of the basal cells to some sort of trauma or inflammation. Keratomas have been found under the sole and frog in a discrete spherical form.

They may not cause lameness, and may only be discovered at a post mortem; if they do cause pain, it is due to their size and position.

As explained above, they are most commonly found down the dorsal wall, but they can develop elsewhere, including the bar. There may be no evidence of a keratoma externally, but sometimes it can be seen under the foot displacing the white line, and may be the cause of recurrent abscesses or be found as the underlying factor for a sandcrack, though this is rare. A keratoma cannot be seen on a radiograph, but often the pressure from it causes bone remodelling, and this is visible.

Treatment involves surgical removal with temporary hoof reconstruction. Most horses will make a full recovery and return to work after the surgery.

NAVICULAR DISEASE

Also known as navicular syndrome, palmar foot pain syndrome, caudal foot lameness.

Historically, 'navicular disease' was used to refer to what was considered to be a degenerative disease of the navicular bone that caused intermittent lameness in the front feet of horses, which could be 'blocked' with a low palmar nerve block, and showed changes in the navicular bone on radiographs. Even before the introduction of magnetic resonance imaging (MRI), it was realized that horses with 'navicular disease' had problems in other structures close to the navicular bone, and because of this, vets started to use the diagnostic term 'navicular syndrome'.

MRI and post-mortem studies have shown that any of the structures that make up the 'navicular apparatus' (*see* Fig. 207) can be involved in this condition, and in most cases, damage in one or more of these other tissues accompanies changes to the navicular bone. Because 'navicular disease' is still more commonly used than 'navicular syndrome', or the even less specific 'palmar foot pain' or 'caudal foot lameness' used by some vets, I will use 'navicular disease' in this text, but emphasize that it can involve damage to any

of the structures 'in the vicinity of the navicular bone', and not just the navicular bone.

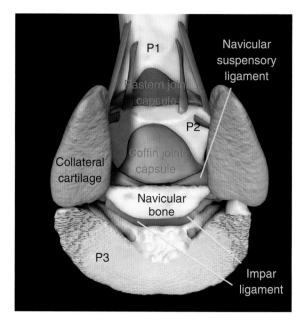

Fig. 208   The DDFT, which passes palmar to the navicular bone to insert on P3, is absent in this image. The main supporting ligaments of the navicular bone are the navicular suspensory ligament (attached to the proximal border) and the impar ligament (on its distal border). The navicular bone also has ligaments to the collateral cartilages and the DDFT. (Image courtesy Science in 3D-the University of Georgia Research Foundation)

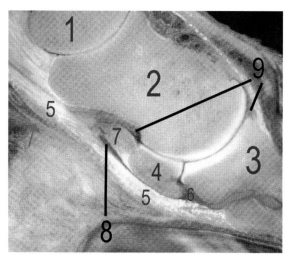

Fig. 207   The structures involved in the navicular apparatus (podotrochlear apparatus), all of which can be involved in 'navicular disease': 1), 2) and 3) = P1, P2 and P3; 4) the navicular bone; 5) the deep digital flexor tendon (DDFT) – closely associated with the flexor (back) surface of the navicular bone; 6) the impar ligament (distal sesamoidean impar ligament) – the ligament that attaches the distal border of the navicular bone to P3; 7) the navicular suspensory ligament – the ligaments that attach the navicular bone to P1; 8) the navicular bursa – the synovial sac between the navicular bursa and the DDFT; 9) coffin joint. The distal digital annular ligament (green arrow) acts as a sling to support all the other structures. (Image courtesy J-M. Denoix, The Distal Limb)

Symptoms

Because of the range of structures that can be involved, there is bound to be variation in the pattern of lameness seen in navicular disease. The 'classical' picture of navicular disease is as a result of degenerative changes occurring in one or more structures, very often involving both front feet, and the symptoms described here will mostly apply to this form of the disease. However, navicular disease can also apply to a unilateral acute lameness from an injury to one individual structure. 'Classical' navicular disease is generally found in 'middle-aged' horses.

There is a suggestion that some breeds are more susceptible to navicular disease: it is seen, for example, more frequently in American Quarter Horses and Warmbloods which tend to have narrower and more upright feet, and in Thoroughbreds with their low hoof angle. However, it may be the type of work that these horses do – repeated intense work – that is the significant factor in causing the degenerative changes.

The foot with a low hoof angle, which may be 'broken back', is blamed for increased loading of the navicular apparatus. For those with upright feet, it is sometimes suggested that navicular pain causes the horse to change its stance to reduce the load on the back of the foot, and this causes the feet to become more narrow and upright. However, I think it is more likely that an upright foot causes 'navicular' changes, from its limited ability to flex and absorb concussion, rather than to result from it.

The following patterns of lameness may indicate that a horse is suffering from navicular disease.

- If affected unilaterally, some horses will change their stance, tending not to fully weight the affected foot and regularly placing it slightly ahead of the other one.
- The pattern of lameness is often intermittent,

settling down but then returning when the horse is back in work.

- Lameness is usually worse when the horse is trotted on hard ground, and more obvious when trotted in a circle with the affected leg on the inside. If both feet are affected, the horse may be lame on one leg when trotted in a circle in one direction and then lame on the other leg when trotted in the other direction.
- It may be thought that the horse is lame in only one leg, but following a nerve block when investigating the lameness, the horse is then found to be also lame on the other front leg.
- Horses that walk with a toe-first landing may well do so because of navicular pain. With navicular disease, it has been demonstrated that the deep flexor muscle contracts and tightens the DDFT earlier in the stance phase than normal, in what seems to be an attempt to limit joint movement and reduce the pain. It may be that the deep flexor muscle is tightened early in anticipation of the pain, before the foot hits the ground, and this could account for the tendency to land toe first. Because toe-landing inevitably shortens the anterior phase of the stride, lameness from navicular disease is sometimes mistaken for a shoulder problem.

There are some simple tests that might help to point to navicular disease, though in themselves they are not diagnostic. Thus, lameness may be worse following a flexion test, where the digit is held firmly in a flexed position for around a minute and the horse then trotted off.

Some people report that in cases of navicular disease, pain can be elicited if firm pressure is applied over the centre of the frog. (This obviously needs to be differentiated from painful conditions of the frog, for example thrush.)

If a horse is stood with a wedge under the toe, tilting the foot back, and then trotted off,

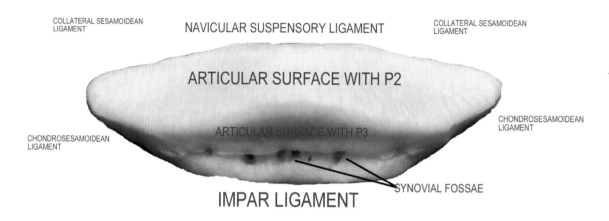

COLLATERAL SESAMOIDEAN LIGAMENT

NAVICULAR SUSPENSORY LIGAMENT

COLLATERAL SESAMOIDEAN LIGAMENT

ARTICULAR SURFACE WITH P2

CHONDROSESAMOIDEAN LIGAMENT

ARTICULAR SURFACE WITH P3

CHONDROSESAMOIDEAN LIGAMENT

SYNOVIAL FOSSAE

IMPAR LIGAMENT

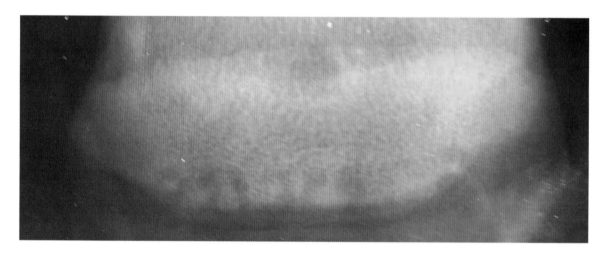

COLLATERAL SESAMOIDEAN LIGAMENT

NAVICULAR SUSPENSORY LIGAMENT

COLLATERAL SESAMOIDEAN LIGAMENT

FLEXOR SURFACE

CHONDROSESAMOIDEAN LIGAMENT

CHONDROSESAMOIDEAN LIGAMENT

IMPAR LIGAMENT

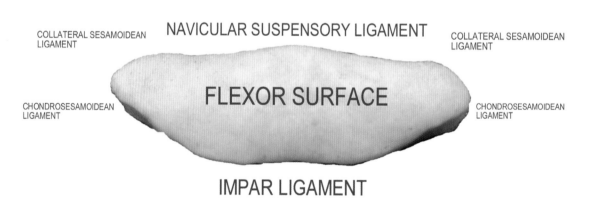

Figs 209 a, b and c   The specimen navicular bone (dorsal and palmar views) is normal and not the one from the radiograph. The multiple dark areas in the navicular bone, particularly of the distal (lower) border, are the changes that are likely to be seen in navicular disease.

some horses with navicular disease become lamer.

Pathology

In the past, trying to work out what caused navicular disease relied on radiography and the study of the end result – the study of clinical cases post mortem. The introduction of MRI now allows the structures of the navicular apparatus to be studied in the live horse, which can provide information about the disease process before the case becomes a cadaver specimen.

The navicular bone is joined to all the other structures of the palmar foot by ligaments. The impar ligament, that attaches the distal border of the navicular bone to P3, is made up of bundles of fibres interspersed with looser connective tissue that contains nerves and also blood vessels that provide about 75 per cent of the navicular bone's blood supply. Where the impar ligament inserts on P3, its fibres blend with those of the DDFT and the synovial membrane as it attaches to the bone. The rest of the blood supply to the navicular bone enters through the dorsal border, through the navicular suspensory ligament. The DDFT is reinforced by a fibrocartilage plaque where it passes palmar to (behind) P2 and the navicular bone.

Studying navicular disease has inevitably concentrated on changes occurring in the navicular bone, because these can be picked up on radiographs, but damage can be found in any of the other structures of the navicular apparatus – for example:

- **In the navicular bone:** Surface changes and deeper erosions on the flexor surface of the navicular bone, fractures of the distal border of the bone, fluid in the bone (seen on MRI), and an increase in the number of, and enlargement of the synovial fossae.

- **Changes in the DDFT:** Splits in the surface of the DDFT, fibre disruption and fibre degeneration as well as adhesions between the navicular bone and the DDFT.
- **Involvement of the navicular bursa:** There can be inflammation and thickening of the navicular bursa, an increase in fluid in the bursa and adhesions can form between the navicular bone and the navicular bursa.
- **In the supporting ligaments of the navicular bone:** Damage and disruption may be found in the impar, suspensory or collateral ligaments.

Several suggestions have been made about what causes the pain in navicular disease, including venous congestion causing increased interosseous (inside the bone) pressure in the navicular bone, distension of the navicular bursa, and with the frequency of damage in the impar and collateral sesamoidean ligaments, pain from the nerve endings in these ligaments.

In some cases there is loss of fibrocartilage on the palmar surface of the navicular bone, accompanied by fibre damage to the DDFT overlying this, but it is not certain which of these changes develops first, or how much of the pain they contribute to. It seems likely that these changes occur in the later stages of the disease, when the horse becomes more persistently lame, and it may be that the horse's protective response, of putting more pressure on the back (palmar surface) of the navicular bone by tightening the tendon, actually compounds the problem.

Diagnosis

Radiographic changes are not uncommonly seen in the navicular bone in apparently sound horses, so a diagnosis of navicular disease from radiographs has to be made with caution. It seems probable that radiographic changes seen in different parts of the navicular bone reflect damage to the ligaments that attach at those sites, and what makes diagnosis difficult is that these bone changes are likely to persist after any tear in the ligament has repaired.

It seems that the more obvious the changes seen in the bone, the more likely they are to be significant, and I think that any vet would consider the changes seen in Fig. 209b to be abnormal. Unfortunately, when many vets see changes to the navicular bone, they seem to find it all too easy to make the diagnosis of navicular disease. The changes in the navicular bone in Fig. 187 prompted a diagnosis of navicular disease, in spite of P3 rotation and the laminar wedge apparent on another radiograph, indicating a chronic laminitis.

A diagnosis of navicular disease still relies on the pattern of lameness, a positive low palmar digital nerve block and radiographic changes, but should only be made when everything else has been ruled out.

Local anaesthetic blocks of the coffin joint, the navicular bursa and the DDFT (sheath), radio-isotope scintigraphy, CT scans, arthroscopy or ultrasonography may all help to confirm a diagnosis of navicular disease, but MRI seems to provide the greatest amount of information about which structures are involved.

Treatment and Management

For very many cases of navicular disease, these further investigations will not be carried out, often due to cost, and horses with navicular disease will be treated empirically as they have been in the past.

Initially, many cases of navicular disease will improve with rest, but the horse becomes lame again when exercise is resumed. Judging how long a horse should be off work without knowing exactly which parts of the navicular apparatus are involved, is extremely difficult for a vet, as well as being extremely frustrating for

an owner, particularly if it turns out to be too short a time and the horse goes lame again. It seems likely that the more times the horse goes lame, the more damage is done, and this can eventually lead to chronic changes that make the horse permanently lame.

The 'traditional' shoe applied for navicular disease is one with a rolled toe and thicker at the heels. These reduce the mechanical forces on the navicular apparatus by reducing the pressure from the DDFT, at rest due to the raised heel and when moving by shortening the breakover. One can understand how this might help the broken-back foot with collapsed heels, by helping to realign the HPA and relieve pain in the area, but it will not achieve much in the long term if the heel collapse is not addressed. For the narrow upright foot, the problem would seem to be the concussive forces concentrated onto a small area that the rigid hoof structure cannot compensate for. In these feet, the bars extend high up inside the foot and it seems reasonable that the horse would tighten the DDF muscle to stop the navicular bone thumping down on top of them at every step. This has prompted the suggestion that the bars be trimmed aggressively, and there seems to be some sense in this because it should allow more hoof movement by reducing the restriction of the back of the foot and allowing the bars to 'escape' from the descending bones.

There are many reports of people dealing with 'navicular disease' successfully without shoes, but I couldn't say whether this is due to being unshod, or the method of trim and the length of time the horse is given to recover.

Without a more specific diagnosis, balancing the feet and trimming the bars, giving a reasonable period of rest, and slowly bringing the horse back into work will hopefully let things settle down.

NSAIDs may be able to settle the problem down early in the disease. At one point, isoxsuprine and warfarin were given for navicular disease when it was believed to be ischaemia (lack of oxygen) in the navicular bone that produced the changes in it, but this theory has been discarded, as, it seems, has this line of treatment. Some vets have started using tiludronic acid as a treatment for navicular disease, and it is given to 'reduce bone resorption' in the navicular bone. The likelihood that this will help to treat navicular disease will presumably depend on which structures are damaged, and the jury is still out as to whether this treatment is effective, or whether it is an expensive way to pass the time while the damaged tissues repair (if it does).

As degenerative changes progress, it becomes more and more difficult to keep the horse sound, and if regular dosing with 'bute' can no longer control it, some vets will resort to cutting the nerves (neurectomy).

COFFIN JOINT DISEASE

Coffin joint disease can be a relatively straightforward inflammation in the coffin joint, causing swelling of the joint capsule with pain and restriction of movement, but at other times more serious changes occur in the joint. Inflammation in a joint (arthritis) causes changes to the synovial membrane which can reduce synovial fluid production, leading to degenerative changes in the cartilage covering the bones, degenerative joint disease (DJD).

The distended joint capsule may be palpable above the coronary band over the dorsal wall. The horse will be lame, and flexion of the lower leg joints is likely to worsen the lameness.

An abaxial sesamoid nerve block or a joint block of the coffin joint are both likely to remove the lameness. When local anaesthetic is injected into the coffin joint, it has been found to reach the navicular bursa, which can make it difficult to differentiate between joint and bursa problems.

The joint can be medicated directly, using corticosteroids and/or hyaluronic acid (normally

present in the joint), and for those cases that have become more chronic, arthroscopic examination of the joint will allow removal of damaged cartilage and debris from the joint.

CONDITIONS OF THE BONE

The common denominators for this group of conditions are as follows.

- They are likely to have lameness as the only symptom.
- The horse is unlikely to go sound after a low palmar nerve block and will require an abaxial-sesamoid nerve block to make it sound.
- Diagnosis can generally be made from radiographs.

BONE FRACTURES

The brittle nature of bones makes them liable to fracture. This can be from external trauma or when a bone is subjected to excessive internal stresses, when these are in a different direction to that which the bone's structure is designed to withstand.

Some fractures of P1 and P2 are the result of direct trauma, but these may also occur with twisting, when foot movement is restricted as the horse turns sharply, from a hole in the ground or possibly due to studs or toe-grabs fitted to the shoe. Hyperextension of the fetlock joint can cause the proximal end of P1 to chip or the suspensory ligament to pull away from the proximal sesamoid bones, taking a piece of bone with it.

P3 has to withstand significant forces, but fractures of it are not common since it is protected by the hoof and by the way the other structures in the foot help to redistribute the forces affecting it. Fractures of P3 are divided into fractures of the body of the bone that involve the joint, which are far more serious, and those that don't, which include fractures of the extensor process, palmar process or the solar border of the bone.

Fractures around the rim of the solar border can be a problem in racehorses, due to their intensive work and their shape of foot, but these are also seen with bone remodelling in cases of chronic laminitis. Chip fractures of the extensor process are likely to occur from hyperextension of the coffin joint.

Symptoms

Whatever the fracture, lameness is likely to be of sudden onset, generally with no other visible signs, although a split along the coronary band may accompany a fracture if caused by the foot striking a solid object.

On examination, pain will probably be elicited by flexion of the coffin joint, if the fracture involves the joint, and when applying pressure using hoof testers in other cases.

Diagnosis of P3 fractures will usually be possible from radiographs, by seeing a dark fracture line through the bone. Radio-isotope scintigraphy, CT scans or MRI may be required to identify fractures in some instances.

Treatment may involve surgery, with screw fixation for fractures involving the joint and for chip removal from avulsion fractures. Other fractures are generally treated by limiting hoof movement, by stabling the horse and using some form of foot cast, or perhaps with a bar shoe with quarter clips, to assist the ready-made splint, the hoof, to stabilize the fracture.

SIDEBONE

Calcification of the collateral cartilages probably results from low grade trauma, from internal rather than external forces, and seems to be more common in horses that land heavily on their feet. Side-bone formation is likely to be in response to stress and imbalance in the foot, but it would be unusual for them to be the cause of lameness unless there is extensive ossification. In these cases, the bone laid down may involve the ligament attachment to the DDFT or the collateral ligaments of the coffin joint, which lie at the front (dorsal) edge of the cartilage. Identification of sidebone is usually done from radiographs, but if extensive ossification is present the rigid proximal border of the cartilage may be palpable.

RINGBONE

Ringbone refers to a situation where extra bone

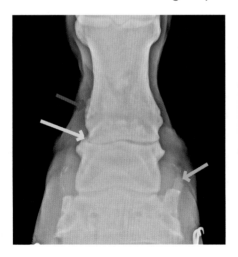

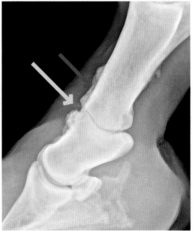

Fig. 210 'High' articular ringbone affecting the pastern joint, with extra bone formed around the joint (blue arrow). Part of the joint has collapsed, with the joint space narrower dorsally and on the medial side of the joint (yellow arrow). There is also some 'sidebone' present (green arrow). (Images courtesy of Joe Rosenberg DVM Paniolo Equine Clinic San Diego California.

is laid down on the phalangeal bones. If it involves a joint it is called 'articular ringbone', and 'non-articular ringbone' when not involving a joint. Articular ringbone is a form of arthritis and usually occurs from abnormal loading of the joint, either due to conformation or the horse's action, and if it involves the pastern joint is referred to as 'high' ringbone, or 'low' ringbone if the coffin joint is affected. When excessive strain is put on to the attachments of the tendons or joint capsule to the bone, the periosteum that covers it is disrupted and responds by producing extra bone.

Most of the joint changes involve the dorsal surface, and from the way the horse tries to reduce the pain, the heels tend to become worn. Horses with ringbone are very likely to react to a flexion test, sometimes finding flexion of the pastern painful, and commonly trotting off more lame after this. Sometimes the pastern bones can feel large on palpation, but diagnosis is usually made from radiographs.

There is not a great deal that can be done for articular ringbone once significant amounts of extra bone have formed, other than making the horse comfortable and slowing the progression of the ringbone. Because the problem most commonly affects the dorsal surface, any trimming or shoeing that changes bone alignment may cause more pain. The aim is to ease the breakover all around the foot, as well as ensuring good medio-lateral balance, but each case can have its own individual requirement to make the horse more comfortable. It is this type of condition that can particularly benefit from the use of leverage testing to assess the most comfortable position for the horse in order to work out the best trim/shoeing protocol for it.

Many horses with ringbone will be managed by giving NSAIDs, and this allows the horse to continue doing light work, which in itself seems to be beneficial. It will also help to keep the weight off a horse, which will reduce the stress on the joint.

Very occasionally, high ringbone is treated surgically, not by removing the extra bone, but by causing more damage to the joint to get it to fuse, thus removing pain from joint movement.

BONE CYSTS

Cysts may be identified on radiographs, and can be discrete inside the bone or may have connection to a joint. These require surgery.

PEDAL OSTEITIS

Pedal osteitis describes inflammatory changes to P3, manifest by changes to the surface or edge of P3 on radiographs. There may be areas of new bone or of bone loss (lysis) on the dorsal surface, the palmar processes or around the perimeter of the bone. Pedal osteitis is likely to be as the result of trauma, often repeated low-grade trauma.

NSAIDs and rest are likely to settle lameness caused by pedal osteitis, but it will recur if the cause of the localized trauma is not addressed.

OSTEOMYELITIS

Osteomyelitis is a bone infection occurring in P3, most commonly from damage from a foreign body or in chronic laminitis when P3 penetrates the sole, and can be diagnosed with radiography. Antibiotics will be given systemically as well as locally, but if this isn't being effective, by applying a tourniquet the bone can be perfused directly by injecting antibiotics into the digital vein.

Sterile maggots are being used to treat solar penetrations, to help remove necrotic (dead) tissue, but surgery may be required to remove infected bone, or a piece of bone that has broken away (a sequestrum), which can act as a foreign body.

12 Investigations, Opinions and Conclusions

Having introduced a number of novel concepts throughout the book, this final chapter gives me the opportunity to provide the background to these ideas and to give an explanation for them. Although this chapter is rather technical, I hope that the knowledge gained from the previous eleven chapters will enable the reader to follow my explanations.

The first part of the chapter follows the path of my investigations that led me to many of my conclusions. A lot of my investigations were done by looking at and measuring the feet of live horses, so owners starting to study horses' feet, through to those who have greater knowledge and who may be skeptical of my observations, can easily do the same research.

No book about horses' feet could ignore the shoeing versus barefoot debate, and this makes up the middle section of the chapter, as well as some more general comments about foot trimming.

In the final section I have attempted to provide an explanation for how the laminae are affected by insulin resistance and how it might trigger laminitis. A lot of what is written in this section is my interpretation of reading research papers and trying to apply the findings to my experiences with IR and laminitis. Although speculative, they do give a possible explanation for why some horses are more likely to develop laminitis, and hopefully will help owners to understand the principles of prevention and management of IR and laminitis in horses and ponies.

ANGLES OF THE FOOT

Dr Pollitt's lectures at the 1998 BEVA Congress, where he presented his novel ideas on the pathogenesis of laminitis (MMP enzymes), made me realize how little I knew about laminitis, and it was after attending a weekend course in 2002, put on by the German vet, Dr

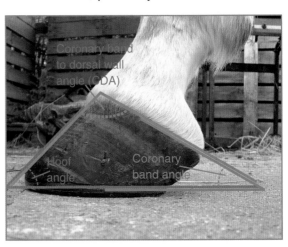

Fig. 211
*Hoof angle = the angle of the dorsal hoof wall to the ground = the angle the **top inch** of the dorsal wall makes with the horizontal (red angle)*

Coronet angle = the angle of the coronary band to the ground = the angle the line joining the coronary band of the dorsal wall to that at the heel bulb makes with the horizontal (green angle)

Coronet to dorsal wall angle (CDA) = the angle of the coronary band to the dorsal wall = the angle the line of the coronary band makes with the top inch of the dorsal wall (purple angle)

Hiltrud Strasser, that I became aware of how little I knew about horses' feet.

As well as making suggestions on all aspects of the management of the horse, the 'Strasser Method' includes advice on the feet and how they should be trimmed. My knowledge of horses' feet was based on 'traditional' theories, and some of these were widely different from those proposed by Dr Strasser. Some of her ideas I agreed with then, and still agree with, some I disagreed with then, and still disagree with, but there were others that I realized I could not give an opinion on because I just didn't know.

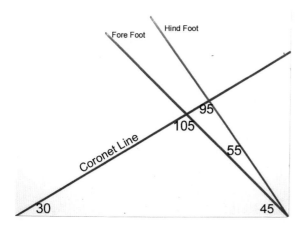

Fig. 212 *The 'PAD', based on the 'Plexiglas' template produced by Sabine Kells for use by Strasser Trimmers, depicting the angles for fore and hind feet. The line at 30 degrees I refer to as the 'coronet line', with the other two, at 45 and 55 degrees (the hoof lines) depicting the line of the dorsal wall of the front feet and hind feet respectively.*

Initially it was Dr Strasser's suggestion that the coronary band to dorsal wall angle (CDA) of front feet was consistently close to 105 degrees that intrigued me. For all the other angles of the foot that are talked and written about, and the disagreement of what these should be, the CDA was an angle that I had never even thought about before, let alone considered that it could be relatively constant.

I made a template similar to that used to trim horses' feet by Strasser trimmers, and started to study the CDA of horses' feet. This was done by lining up the coronet line on the PAD with the hairline of the dorsal wall and the hairline of the bulb of the heel, and then seeing whether the line of the top inch of the dorsal hoof wall coincided with the hoof line at 105 degrees (or 95 degrees for hinds). I was surprised to find that the CDA was close to the suggested 105-degree angle in about 80 per cent of front feet.

Those that did not fit would commonly have a CDA closer to 95 degrees, and this included foals' feet, which had a consistently higher hoof angle than adults, as well as around 10–15 per cent of adult front feet.

· One aspect of the 'Strasser trim' is to trim front feet to a 45-degree hoof angle, which is suggested to give P3 a zero palmar angle (ground-parallel), and if trimmed to this angle, the coronary band angle would be 30 degrees since the sum of the three angles must add up to 180 degrees [45 + 105 + 30 = 180]. For hind feet, with the higher bone angle of 55 degrees and a CDA of 95 degrees, the coronet angle would also be 30 degrees [55 + 95 + 30 = 180]

In a study to assess Strasser's angles, measurement of the hoof and the coronet angle of the front feet of horses attending two veterinary clinics over a two-year period, showed a difference to those suggested by Dr Strasser, with a hoof angle mean (average) of 52.38 degrees instead of 45 degrees, and a coronet angle mean of 23.31 degrees instead of 30 degrees. However, by subtracting these two figures from 180 degrees, this produces an average for the CDA of 104.31 degrees, very close to 105 degrees.

In a more recent study of 300 lame horses, the mean hoof angle was 52.27 degrees and the mean coronet angle 23.13 degrees, which made the mean CDA 104.6 degrees. These figures give some credence to my observations, that the CDA is around 105 degrees, and that there is an inverse relationship between the hoof angle and coronet angle, so that if the hoof angle is 45 degrees plus x degrees, then the coronet-to-ground angle is 30 degrees minus x degrees. (It must be remembered that in both studies these were 'mean' – average – figures, and give no indication of individual variability.)

Using the PAD became a routine for me when looking at all horses' feet. I would check the CDA, but could also assess the hoof angle by placing the PAD on the ground beside the foot. By comparing the line of the top inch of the dorsal wall to the two hoof lines I found:

- The range of hoof angles of the front feet was between 45 and 60 degrees (with very few outside this range), with a large percentage between 50 and 55 degrees (*see* Chapter 4).
- Horses with upright front feet, standing evenly, would almost invariably 'stand under', and not in the 'normal' stance described in books (*see* Chapter 3).
- Horses appeared to be able to alter their stance through a range of hoof angles to maintain a straight HPA, but beyond this they were either broken back or broken forward (*see* Chapter 3).
- There was far greater consistency in the way that farriers and trimmers trimmed the hind feet, close to a 55-degree hoof angle (*see* Chapter 5).

My observation that horses with relatively upright front feet generally stand under did not fit with the commonly used description of the 'normal stance', even though the higher hoof angles were also suggested as being normal.

I identified two situations where attempts made to provide uniformity probably failed to do so. In many research studies of conformation and kinematics, the protocol often states that the feet have been 'trimmed by an experienced farrier to provide a straight HPA', or something similar. The intention is obviously to try to produce conformity of hoof angle for the study, but because the horse is able to change its stance, horses with a wide range of hoof angles could have been included in the studies.

TRIM TO A ZERO PALMAR ANGLE?

Dr Strasser's suggestion that all horses' front feet should be trimmed to give P3 a zero palmar angle (ground-parallel) I believe is wrong. I agree with the proposition that the forces on the laminae around the foot are evenly spread when P3 is in this position, but if trimmed to produce this position at rest, the greater forces of movement and of carrying a rider will cause P3 to tilt backwards to produce a reverse angle. This will unevenly load the laminae, but worse than this will be the abnormal loading of the structures of the palmar foot.

The hoof should be trimmed with P3 having a positive palmar angle so that, when the foot is maximally loaded, P3 will not go beyond ground-parallel and end up with a negative palmar angle.

Factors that might affect this are the shape of the foot, the strength of the hoof horn, the type of work, the speed of work, the ground conditions and the load that the horse carries. In cases suffering with laminitis, the horse will not be working or carrying a rider. In these cases the hoof can be trimmed to give a lower palmar angle, and in bad cases of laminitis, a ground-parallel P3 is not only acceptable but probably necessary.

The other situation is when radiographs are taken with the horse's foot placed on a block with the cannon perpendicular. Positioning an upright foot this way will inevitably make it appear to have a broken-forward HPA, but it might not if the horse were allowed to take its normal stance. I therefore began to question opinions given on bone alignment from radiographs.

Having found that the CDA was, in the majority of cases, around 105 degrees, I needed to know how this related to P3. This required me to investigate another of Dr Strasser's proposals, that the bone angle of P3 was 45 degrees for fores and 55 degrees for hinds. This I did by measuring the P3 bone angle directly on bone specimens, from photographs of bone specimens, and on radiographs. At first glance the bones appeared to have diverse shapes and a range of bone angles, but there seemed to be several reasons for this.

- In order to make an accurate measurement of the bone angle, it has to be assessed at right angles to a level bone, and on many of the photographs and radiographs P3 was tilted.
- A lot of the differences were with the shape of the extensor process, the extent of calcification of the lateral cartilages, and the shape of the tip of P3.
- Very often neither the front edge of the bone nor the solar border was straight. Depending on which parts of the dorsal edge and solar border were measured, there was a range of bone angles that P3 could potentially be given.
- If the dorsal surface line is taken over the central part of the bone and the remodelled periphery ignored, there is much greater uniformity of bone angle than at first glance, with the bone angle close to 45 degrees in most cases.

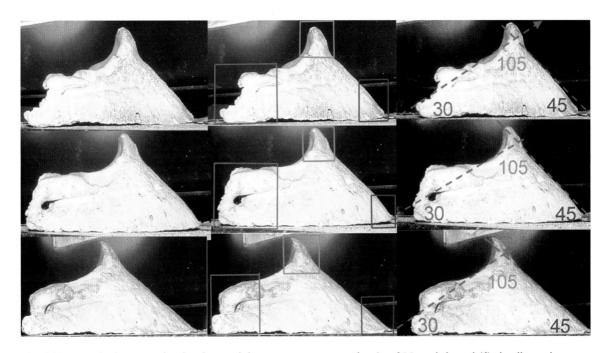

Fig. 213   For the bone angle, the shape of the extensor process, the tip of P3 and the calcified collateral cartilages can be ignored. If the bone angle is measured using the straight area of the dorsal surface below the extensor process relative to the solar border, as it appears on a flat surface, the angle becomes relatively consistent at around 45 degrees.

Having found a relatively consistent bone angle, I wanted to know how the coronary band angle and the CDA related to P3. I found that a line drawn to include the proximal point of the palmar process and the centre of the articular surface of P3, when extended,

---

THE METRON SYSTEM

One of the advantages of digital x-ray equipment is the inclusion of software that can be used to measure features on radiographs. The Metron System is one of these, and I mention this system specifically because it can also be used to mark up photographs, and independent studies have been carried out to verify the accuracy of the measurements obtained from it. By including a marker of known length in the radiograph or photograph, the Metron System can use this for calibration so that any lengths measured will be accurate.

However, the accuracy of distances and angles (using any system) does depend on correct positioning, by the operator, of the foot in relation to the x-ray beam, as well as correct identification and precise marking of the lines and points to be measured.

---

made an angle with the ground of around 30 degrees, and was close to 105 degrees to the dorsal surface of P3 (*see* Fig. 213). So it appeared that there were two concentric triangles based around the centre of mass of P3, in the shape of the bone and in the hoof surrounding it.

HOOF STRENGTH

As well as measuring the hoof angles, I would

also regularly take photographs of the feet. After I had photographed the feet of over a thousand horses and ponies, I hoped to be able to identify individual breed characteristics, but my attempts to do so were limited by the number of cross-breeds and because I had only one or two examples of some breeds. However, this was when I started to recognize differences in hoof shape, and the way that they deformed, which seemed to be directly related to hoof strength (*see* Chapter 4 for a pattern of deformity). Looking at feet in this way, it appeared that hoof form attributed to particular foot conditions might in fact be the *cause* of the problem rather than the result of it.

- The feet of offspring of a cross between a Thoroughbred and any other breed were stronger and generally had less deformity than the pure Thoroughbred.
- There was a pattern to those fore feet whose CDA did not conform to 105 degrees.
- Fore feet that had a CDA of less than 105 degrees were relatively strong feet with high heels combined with a long toe. It appeared that the lack of heel movement did not allow the foot to compensate for the forces on the long toe, which then caused the dorsal wall to curve inwards below the extensor process to produce a lower CDA.
- If laminitis occurs in these feet, the dorsal wall is no longer held by the laminae, so can straighten, and the CDA reverts to 105 degrees. For this reason, the CDA in horses with chronic laminitis is more consistent than in non-laminitic feet!
- Hind feet that appeared to have a CDA greater than 95 degrees were those that had a 'bull-nose' shape, with the heels having some degree of collapse and the dorsal wall convex, but the top inch of growth of the dorsal wall was still around 95 degrees (*see* Chapter 5).

STUDIES OF CADAVER SPECIMENS

The Bars

Another line of investigation I followed related to the significance that Dr Strasser attributed to the bars in the foot, with their effect on hoof movement and blood flow, and how they might contribute to foot problems.

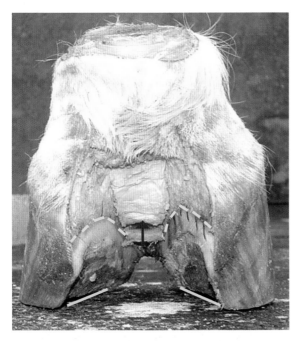

Fig. 214   The frog has been removed from this cadaver specimen of a chronic laminitis case with obvious medio-lateral imbalance. This has exposed the full extent of the bars (proximal border dotted yellow line and distal border solid yellow line). The DDFT has been cut (cut surface between red dotted lines) to identify the position of the navicular bone (blue arrow).

By removing the frog to expose the bars, I noted how easy it was to underestimate the extent of the bars from external examination of the feet, and that, moving forward from the heels, their length typically increased initially before they tapered down to blend into the sole. (For the role of the bars and their importance, *see* Chapters 2 and 6.)

The Relationship of External and Internal Features in a Foot

Whether just assessing foot form, or working out a trimming protocol for a particular foot, there are a number of external features used as markers, by farriers, to provide information about the relative position of the internal structures of the foot. I was interested to know how accurate these might be in different shapes of foot, so started to examine cadaver specimens, as well as looking at other dissection studies.

Angles

Hoof and bone angles are independent of foot size, length of growth or any magnification on a radiograph, but are dependent on the foot position, in relation to the x-ray beam or camera, and the points on the hoof or bone used to make up the angles. (Mid-line sections of cadaver specimens do not include the palmar processes of P3, thus the bone angle cannot be measured. The angle of this central part of the bone appears to be about 10 degrees less than the bone angle that includes the palmar processes.)

If the dorsal hoof wall is straight, the dorsal angle of P3 is close to the hoof angle. When there is deviation of the dorsal wall, the proximal inch of wall is a good reflection of the dorsal angle of P3 if the CDA is 105 degrees – for example in chronic laminitics – but if the CDA is less than 100 degrees, the dorsal angle of P3 is usually closer to that of the distal part of the wall.

Earlier in the chapter I proposed that the three external angles reflected the shape of P3. I also suggested that if the hoof angle was 45 degrees + x degrees, then the coronary band

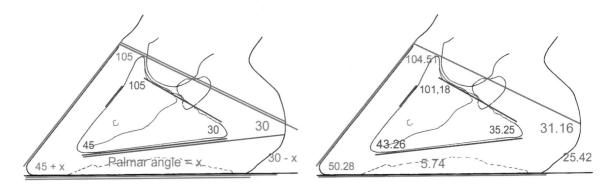

Figs. 215a and b   This diagram was drawn from a radiograph, identified as a 'normal adult foot'. (a) Shows the proposed concentric triangles of the hoof and P3. Not surprisingly, for most feet these angles will be different and (b) shows the actual angles on the diagram. Hoof angle = 45 + 5.28 degrees, coronary band angle = 30 − 4.58 degrees, and the actual palmar angle (×) is 5.74 degrees. The other angle given in purple is that between the coronary band and the solar border of P3.

angle would be 30 − x degrees, in which case, a 30-degree angle to the line of the coronary band should give an indication of the line of the solar border of P3, and the angle this makes with the ground (the palmar angle) would be x degrees (Fig. 215a). However, it is not as straightforward as this, and even in 'normal' feet with a straight dorsal wall and intact laminar attachment, some variation in the angles will be seen. This may be for a variety of reasons.

It may be due to deformation of P3 in the individual horse. Also the angles will vary depending on which parts of the hoof and bone are measured. Thus a photograph taken at right angles to the hairline of the dorsal wall will identify the CDA most accurately, but the ground border of the hoof will be a curved line

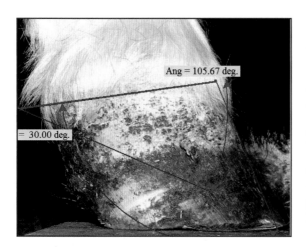
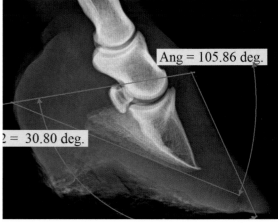

Fig. 216   Because no markers were applied to the feet when the radiograph and photograph were taken, it is not possible to identify accurately the line of the coronary band from these images. (The estimated lines of the coronary band used on these images are within 5 degrees of each other – the Metron System was used to produce the angle measurements).

on the picture, making it impossible to measure the hoof angle accurately.

A radiograph needs to be taken at the level of the solar border of P3 to provide the most accurate measurement of the bone angle and palmar angle. If taken from a higher position, the solar border is less likely to be a straight line, and the palmar processes of P3 will no longer overlie each other.

The proposed angles will still generally apply when there is deviation of the hoof wall in chronic laminitis, provided angles are measured using the proximal dorsal wall.

If the CDA is obviously less than 105 degrees, the proposed angles will no longer apply, but it would appear that the smaller CDA is accompanied by a higher hoof angle and the coronary band angle is not altered, producing a hoof angle of 45 + x + y degrees, CDA of 105 – y degrees, and coronary band angle of 30 – x degrees. It seems that deviation of the dorsal wall does not affect the relationship between P3 and the line of the coronary band.

VERIFICATION NEEDED

The consistency of the angles I have presented has not been verified, and this will need to be done before the use of the PAD can be advocated as an accurate indicator of the palmar angle of P3. While some studies seem to confirm my observations, others do not, but in the text I have identified possible reasons for this.

Using the PAD to Identify the Palmar Angle

It is one thing to suggest to people to use the PAD to study horses' feet, but quite another to advocate that they use it to identify the palmar angle.

Without doubt, the best way to identify the palmar angle is from correctly positioned radiographs, but in the absence of these, I have no doubt that the PAD is the next best thing. The 'PAD', based on the 'Plexiglas' template used by Strasser trimmers, was given its alternative title by a colleague/friend of mine from the acronym for 'palmar angle determiner', this potentially being its most functional use. This, I believe, is applicable in most fore feet, and also in hind feet where it is useful in identifying a negative palmar angle, but experience is needed to be able to interpret the cases where the angles do not fit. The PAD is probably of greatest benefit in cases of chronic laminitis.

The PAD is used in the following way:

- Line up the 'coronet line' of the PAD with the coronary band (the hairline at the dorsal wall to the hairline at the bulb of the heel). Draw a line on the hoof following the bottom edge of the PAD: this marked line will be close to the angle of the solar border of P3, thus giving an indication of the palmar angle.
- Apply barium paste (or a taped-on metal marker) to the dorsal wall and to the bulb of

Fig. 217
Thoroughbred right fore. Metal markers were applied to the skin of the pastern to identify the hair-line at the dorsal wall and at the bulb of the heel. Using the Metron System, I have drawn a line 30 degrees to this coronet line, which is very close to the line of the solar border of P3.

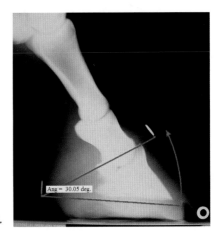

Ang = 30.05 deg.

the heel, to accurately identify the hairline; it should be visible on both a photograph and a radiograph. (Ask your vet to apply markers to the foot when taking radiographs of your laminitis case).

- If a radiograph is taken at the level of the solar border of P3, and a photograph is taken from the same position, the relative accuracy of the estimated (PAD) and true (radiograph) palmar angle can be judged. Provided there is no gross distortion or bone remodelling, the angles are likely to be similar.

- Likewise, the CDA can be measured directly with the PAD or from the photograph, and compared with the radiograph to judge whether it is a good indicator of the dorsal angle of the bone.

- If they are close, it should be possible to use the PAD as a guide for trimming as the case progresses, rather than needing, and having the expense of, repeated radiographs (*see* Figs 55 and 216).

- The PAD should be used as an aid to trimming, rather than as a template for the trim, and the information it provides should help a farrier or trimmer trim to whatever their particular protocol is.

The Sole View

Because the hoof shape is a reflection of the shape of P3 inside it, features closer to the centre of P3, where there is least deformity, will be more accurate than those further from it, from re-modelling of the bone or deformation of the hoof. For this reason, the features of the solar surface used as guides for foot assessment and for trimming are based around the centre of the foot, in the midline and/or between the central cleft and apex of the frog.

Duckett's Dot is a point on the frog ¾in palmar to its apex that has been used as a reference point for over a hundred years (Professor William Russell) but received its

---

CONFUSION IN TERMINOLOGY

The 'centre of rotation' of the coffin joint is the point in the distal condyle of P2 around which the coffin bone (P3) rotates (this is the mathematical definition): the brown dot on Fig. 218.

The 'centre of articulation' (articulation = joint) is the centre of the coffin joint: the green cross on Fig. 218.

Unfortunately both terms are used to refer to each point by different people.

The 'centre of mass' (or centre of balance) of P3 is the point in the bone where if placed in any orientation on a pin the bone would balance: the black dot on Fig. 218.

---

catchy name from studies carried out by the farrier David Duckett (also the source of other terms now in common use, such as 'pillars' at the toe quarters and '(frog) bridge' underneath the navicular bone). It is suggested that a vertical line through Duckett's Dot passes through the insertion of the DDFT, the centre of mass of P3, and the insertion of the extensor tendon (*see* Fig. 218).

The widest part of the foot refers to the widest part of the sole, and a line drawn across the foot to identify this is generally about an inch behind the frog apex. There is a suggested relationship between the widest part of the foot and centre of rotation of the coffin joint and the tip of P3.

Any distance measurements used to indicate a positional relationship between internal and external features will vary with the size of the foot and/or the length of growth, the hoof angle and magnification on radiographs. As the foot grows, those parts of the foot in front of the centre of P3 will move forwards, away from it, and the surface structures in the back part of the foot will grow more towards it, which must affect their relationship to the internal

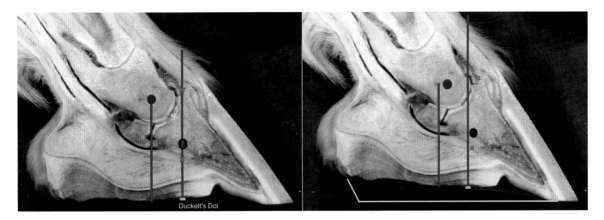

Fig. 218 It is suggested that a vertical line through Duckett's Dot passes through the centre of mass of P3 (black dot) and the DDFT and digital extensor tendon insertions (red crosses). With a 5-degree increase in palmar angle, the line still passes through the broad insertion of the DDFT but is palmar to the centre of the bone and the insertion of the extensor tendon.
The relationship of the centre of rotation of the coffin joint to a fixed point on the frog will also be altered by changes in hoof angle.

Brown dot = the 'centre of rotation' of the coffin joint
Black dot = the 'centre of mass' of P3
Green cross = the 'centre of articulation' of the coffin joint
Yellow cross = the centre of the articular surface of P3

structures. These factors have to be taken into consideration when using these external points of reference.

Further Observations on Hoof Structures

Sometimes I dissected feet to study a particular feature or problem, but in other cases I found changes that stimulated new thoughts and ideas.

The 'Ledge'

It was the laminitic foot (*see* Fig. 142) with such an obvious 'ledge' that no longer supported the tip of P3, which had rotated, which made me think about the support that this rim of sole provided. Any reason for the wall to move away from P3 leaves the edge of the bone resting on more flexible sole than the slightly

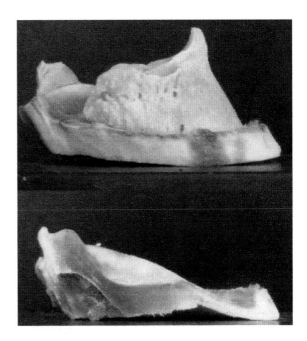

Fig. 219 P3 has lost its support from the ledge, and its tip pressing on weaker sole has allowed P3 to descend. A dissected specimen by Mike Savoldi.

thicker rim of sole with its added stability from the adjoining wall. This was most obvious in cases of laminitis, but could also be seen when there was flaring of the wall for other reasons. These observations might be summarized as follows.

- In chronic laminitis, the tip of P3 rests on unsupported sole (*see* Fig. 143).
- It seemed to be an explanation for the 'distal descent' of P3 in flared feet.
- Certainly in some cases, the 'toe callous' was not thickened sole but more prominent sole of normal thickness (*see* Chapter 6).
- The effect of the distal toe flare in club feet, and the tip of the 'foal foot' flaring from the 'new' hoof, cause the tip of the bone to lose its support (*see* Chapter 5).
- When the tip of P3 is resting on the sole and not on the 'ledge', horses will be more uncomfortable on hard and uneven ground.

The Cycle of Growth of the Horn Structures

Seeing the layers in the sole (*see* Fig. 36) started me thinking about the cyclical growth of the hoof structures. The layers of sole and frog, and the growth lines on the hoof wall, all seem to point to a brief break in growth, which can provide a 'safety mechanism' for the foot. If these structures just kept growing without a break, the foot could only rely on wear to prevent it from becoming overgrown, which would reduce the hoof's ability to expand and contract and limit its ability to absorb concussion. A grossly thickened frog would also limit its sensory role. Having the ability to shed any excess sole, in layers, allows extra wall to break away, and because the break in hoof growth follows the shape of the coronary groove, the harder outer wall can break off while leaving the sensitive dermis still covered by the more flexible inner wall (*see* Fig. 220).

THE SHOEING DEBATE

One cannot write a book about horses' feet without, at some point, discussing the use of horseshoes. Farriers know that metal shoes and nails cause damage to the hoof structure, but

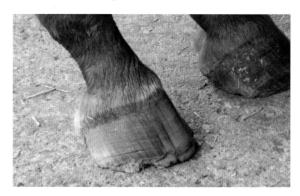

Fig. 220   If the hoof wall becomes overgrown, it generally breaks away along the weak line where there was a break in growth, rather than tearing the whole wall away from the dermis.

argue that they are a 'necessary evil', whereas those in the barefoot movement feel they are an 'unnecessary evil'. The introduction of horseshoes of materials other than metal which have alternative methods of fixing them to the foot, as well as advances in the design of hoof boots, reduces the 'necessity' of the metal shoe; but rightly or wrongly, their relatively low cost and ease of application means that they are likely to continue to be the common 'footwear' for the working horse.

The way that the equid's feet are able to adapt to different living environments is one of the reasons why equids (horses, donkeys and zebra) have survived. But the requirements of domesticated horses, and the unnatural conditions in which many of them are maintained, mean that their feet are less capable of coping with the demands on them, thus increasing the need for some form of foot protection.

Horses and ponies not in work – such as foals, brood mares, 'companion animals' and 'pasture pets' – are unlikely to require any form of protection. For working horses and ponies, whether they need protection (or not) will depend on how strong the hooves are, whether they are 'conditioned' for the surface the horse is being worked on (see 'Soles' in Chapter 6), and the intensity and frequency of the work they are doing.

The reality is that the environmental conditions and the boarding situations in which many owners keep their horses make it difficult to maintain them barefoot, which is why, in the UK, the normal practice still is to have the horse shod once it starts to work, and to carry on shoeing it until it retires. The resurgence of the barefoot movement has caused more owners to question whether their horse or pony needs to be shod, rather than having shoes put on because 'it is the thing to do', and with the increase in the alternatives now available, the number of horses being kept without shoes seems to be on the increase. The benefits of keeping the horse barefoot are:

- Lack of nail damage
- Reduced damage to structures from vibration
- Preventing hoof deformity caused directly by shoeing
- Having better 'hoof function' without the restriction of the nailed-on shoe
- The feet can be trimmed more frequently, particularly when trying to correct a deformity
- Reduced peripheral loading (less of a problem in the shod foot on soft ground)
- The difference in the cost of trimming (plus the cost of hoof-boots) versus the cost of shoeing.

These benefits have to be weighed up against the following disadvantages:
- The extra commitment required to condition the feet in a wet environment (not so critical if boots are used)

- The increased frequency of abscesses in wet conditions. The softer horn structures are less resilient and more prone to sole splits and wall cracks from stone damage, against which shoes provide some protection
- The availability of a suitable trimmer (or farrier)
- Although shoe loss is greater in muddy conditions, nailed-on shoes will generally stay on better than any of the alternatives.

Further benefits of metal shoes are that a pad fitted under a shoe can help to protect the sole, or can provide sole support when dental impression material is put under it. A 'hospital plate' on the ground surface of a shoe can help to protect and manage some injuries, diseases or surgical wounds on the bearing surface of the foot. Fitting studs can help improve traction, and shoes can provide hoof stability when this is needed, for example to help P3 fractures to repair and to limit hoof movement; they can also provide a base for repair material when dealing with hoof cracks. Different designs and positioning of a shoe can be used to alter a horse's action or foot placement, sometimes to help injuries higher up the limb to heal.

IR horses with low grade laminitis can be more footsore on uneven and stony ground, and shoeing can help some of these horses by allowing them to be more regularly exercised, thus helping to keep IR under control. Support can be supplied to the frog or sole to help prevent the detrimental effect of peripheral loading in these cases.

Some of the damage caused by shoeing can be reduced by using shoes of different materials than metal, and some of the difficulties of keeping a horse barefoot, or the problems dealt with by shoes, can be overcome with the use of hoof-boots, the quality of which is improving all the time: they are easier to fit, they stay on better, traction is improved and they are less likely to rub.

FOOT TRIMMING

Many farriers will trim a barefoot horse in the same way that they trim a foot to apply a shoe, with a flat bearing surface all around the wall. This 'pasture trim' will generally be adequate for horses just out on pasture, but is unlikely to be suitable for the working horse. Over the past twenty years, the way barefoot horses are trimmed has changed, based on protocols suggested by a number of people, most notably Jaime Jackson, Dr Hiltrud Strasser, Gene Ovnicek, K. C. La Pierre and Pete Ramey, with contributions from several other farrier-turned-barefoot advocates. Most of these protocols are based on the shape of wild horses' feet, and are provided with physiological and mechanical explanations of the benefits of trimming to this shape.

Although I agree with much of what the 'authors' of these protocols suggest, some followers of their methods have become as single-minded in their approach as the more 'traditional' farrier is about his. I suggest that trimming all feet in the same way is as unsuitable as applying the same type of shoe to every foot.

Studies of feral horses have identified different lengths and shapes of feet of horses in different environments, which some will consider an adaptive process, but many of the differences will be purely the result of an altered balance between growth and wear. The small, rounded feet of horses living on stony and hard ground would sink into a soft substrate and make it difficult for them to move around in these conditions, whereas the overgrown, spread feet of horses living on this surface cope with it far better because the greater surface area of the feet reduces the amount they sink into it and allows them to push against the soft surface when they move. If these horses swop living environments, the reduced wear of the rounded hoof allows it to spread, and the overgrown hoof breaks away

or is worn down to provide feet better suited to their new environment.

There is, of course, a difference between a horse surviving in the wild and one being ridden and remaining sound, many of the reasons having been mentioned above under shoeing. As well as considering what the 'correct' trim or shoe for the individual horse's action, conformation and foot form might be (*see* Chapter 3), we need to take into account the environment the horse lives in and the ground conditions it works on. If we round off the feet to resemble those of a mustang, we cannot expect a horse to run so fast or to manoeuvre so well if it is working on soft ground. If we leave the wall long and work the horse on hard surfaces, the horse's action will be affected by the delayed breakover, possibly causing stress and strain on other parts of the leg or body, and the hooves may break away or be more liable to deform.

Observations on Trimming

The foot has its own methods of limiting overgrowth, which may be suitable for a wild horse in its environment, but are more likely to result in problems in the domesticated horse living and working on different surfaces. In this situation, the hoof is likely to need trimming to remove excess growth, to balance the foot and to reduce forces contributing to deformation.

It has been proposed that feet should be trimmed (or shod) so that a vertical line from the centre of rotation should be close to the midpoint of the foot (or shoe). Studying radiographs, I found this never to be the case, and the dorso-palmar ratio was never less than 55:45 per cent, was more commonly 60:40 per cent, and in some instances was even more. The ratio was worst when the hoof was longer, particularly if the heels were collapsed and growing forwards, and in every case would be improved by trimming. The further forward the toe is from the centre of rotation, the greater forces there will be on the dorsal wall when the horse's foot breaks over.

Although the wear on the feet of wild horses in arid conditions keeps them short, and the rounded edge, particularly at the toe, will produce a bearing surface of the foot closer to 50:50 per cent, this mid-point ratio has not been achieved on any of the (few) radiographs of these feet that I have seen. If the ratio in these 'natural' feet is not 50:50, why should we be trying to trim and shoe horses to these parameters?

It seems to me that a better relationship would be for the ground surface of the hoof to be balanced under the centre of mass of P3, so that the load is evenly spread around the whole foot. Radiographs seem to confirm this, quite often showing a 50:50 per cent ratio to this point in the trimmed foot. However, this relates to static loading rather than loading when the horse is moving.

Bringing the breakover point back on a foot (hoof or shoe) will be of greatest benefit for horses on dry, hard ground particularly for feet

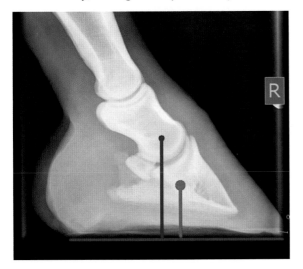

Fig. 221 *Right fore of a barefoot eventer. The perpendicular line from the centre of rotation of the coffin joint has a ground surface ratio of 56:44 per cent (dorsal to palmar), whereas that from the centre of P3 is 50:50 per cent.*

with a lower hoof angle (the protocol trim for a Natural Balance shoe). It will help to reduce the forces on the dorsal wall, so will be beneficial in cases of laminitis (and low grade laminitis), as well as making it easier to correct a hoof deformity.

It will be less suitable in wetter environments, since a foot that rolls over very easily will reduce the horse's ability to push off in soft ground. The weaker spread foot of the thoroughbred in a perimeter shoe may help the horse to run faster on this surface, but the increased forces on their weaker feet are more likely to cause hoof distortion.

The following general considerations should be observed regarding trimming.

- Keeping a well balanced, 'normal' foot in shape is far easier than trying to correct a deformed one.
- Correction of hoof deformities will be easier if the interval between trimmings is shorter
- Monitor changes in response to trimming/ shoeing methods – keeping a photographic record of the feet will help in this.
- Take time to consider the requirements of the horse and its environment: if it is living and working on different surfaces, trim/shoe it for its working environment.

When assessing the foot, always look for evidence of IR, such as obvious hoof rings and a widened white line. Identify the deformity – marking the foot or using the PAD can be helpful. Check the ratio of the ground-bearing surface of the foot in front and behind Duckett's Dot, ¾in (19mm) behind the apex of the frog. Check the ratio of the ground-bearing surface of the foot in front and behind the widest part of the foot

As well as the DDFT that passes palmar to it, the navicular bone is supported by the bars and the fibrous (or fibrocartilage) band that joins the two collateral cartilages. This band, sometimes referred to as the 'frog bridge', is just in front of

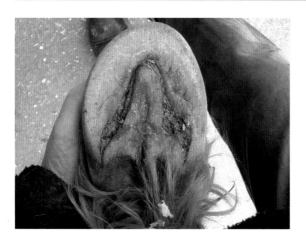

Fig. 222 The closest I could find (in the UK) to a 'wild mustang' foot (hind foot). This Welsh Cob stallion had attention from the farrier 'every six months whether he needed it or not'.

the central cleft of the frog, and the navicular bone lies just dorsal to the anterior edge of the bar laminae. Taking into consideration foot shape and length, these two external features can give an indication of the position of the navicular bone.

If the heels are trimmed to the widest part of the frog (to the level where the hoof blends with the frog), P3 will be very close to ground-parallel (zero palmar angle). The more the heels extend beyond this, the higher the palmar angle will be. (*See* Chapter 6 for comments about bar, sole and frog trimming.)

When barefoot, there are some possible alterations to the simple 'pasture trim' that might be suitable:

'Quarter relief': This involves trimming slightly more hoof from the quarters to leave a slight curvature to the bearing surface of the hoof in this area. This will allow greater movement of the heels on harder ground, but needs the bars to provide support to the heels otherwise it can lead to further heel collapse.

'Toe callous': This refers to a prominent sole

seen just behind the white line, and it should not be touched. Removing any sole here will reduce protection and/or support.

'Mustang roll': A term coined by Jaime Jackson to refer to rounding the edge of the hoof, so it is similar to that found on wild mustangs living on hard terrain. However, for the domestic horse in wet environments, too great a roll on the wall can leave a weakened 'ledge', which reduces the support to the periphery of the bone, and will also limit traction.

LAMINITIS: SOME FINAL THOUGHTS

Despite a great deal of research, a unifying cause of laminitis still eludes us. Insulin resistance would appear to be the most likely candidate for this, and metabolic changes appear to play some part in the majority of cases of laminitis.

A Possible Explanation for the Involvement of IR in Laminitis

In 1998, Dr Chris Pollitt presented an explanation for laminitis developing following carbohydrate (grain) overload (CHO) involving the activation of enzymes (matrix metalloproteinase enzymes – MMPs), which was widely accepted as the mechanism in these cases, but did not explain how laminitis was caused by other triggers.

Some of Dr Pollitt's early investigations involved using small pieces of hoof, referred to as 'explants', to try to identify what could cause separation of the laminae. The explants were maintained in a medium (fluid containing nutrients to keep the tissues alive), and different substances were added to this to see if they could cause separation of the laminae.

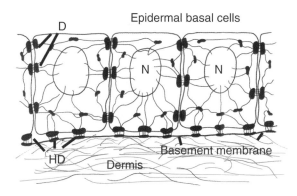

Epidermal basal cells

Fig. 223   The integrity of the basal cell layer relies on the attachments between basal cells (D = desmosome), their attachment to the basement membrane (HD = hemidesmosome), and on the internal cytoskeleton of keratin fibres that connect the desmosomes, hemidesmosomes and the cell nucleus. (N = cell nucleus).

Separation was achieved by adding to the medium an MMP activator that activated the MMPs naturally present in the hoof tissue; however, separation failed to occur when he added a whole range of substances that had been suggested as possible causes of laminitis at the time. The only other situation that did result in separation was when he added something that prevented glucose uptake by the explant. Although separation occurred at the same site, at the basement membrane between the horny and sensitive laminae, the changes in the laminae were found to be different from those produced by enzyme activation.

What are the Changes Found in the Laminae?

Before investigating laminar separation, we should first describe laminar attachment. The basement membrane between the hoof and the sensitive laminae is continuous from the top to the bottom of the hoof and all the way around it, and is firmly attached to the dermis and to the innermost cells of the hoof, the epidermal

basal cells that completely line the secondary epidermal lamellae.

The sites of attachment of basal cells to the basement membrane are called 'hemidesmosomes', and where the cells attach to each other are called 'desmosomes' (*see* Fig. 223). Inside the basal cells there is a network of keratin fibres that connect the cell nucleus to the desmosomes and hemidesmosomes, as well as these attachment sites to one another, thus providing a strong internal cell skeleton (cytoskeleton). The sheet of basal cells relies on the strength of their attachments to the basement membrane and each other, as well as the cytoskeleton, to maintain their shape under tension and to effectively spread the tensile forces that the laminae are subjected to.

When laminar separation is caused by glucose deprivation in explants, the basement membrane is not directly affected and it is the basal cell layer where breakdown occurs. The strength of this layer of cells is reduced by the loss of the desmosome and the hemidesmosome attachments, as well as the disappearance of the keratin fibres of the internal cytoskeleton. The cells lose their

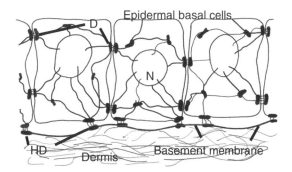

Epidermal basal cells

Fig. 224   D = desmosome, HD = hemidesmosome, N = cell nucleus. The basal cell layer is weakened by the loss of desmosomes, hemidesmosomes and the loss of cytoskeleton. The cells lose their uniform shape, and the cell nuclei change shape and become displaced. A much smaller mechanical force is needed to cause these attachments to break down and separation of the laminae to occur.

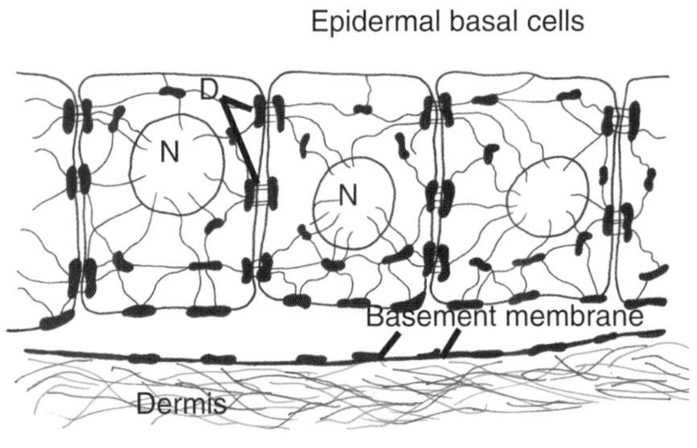

Epidermal basal cells

Fig. 225 When an MMP-activator was added to explants that were not under tension, the glycoprotein filaments that attach the basement membrane to the basal cells in the hemidesmosomes were broken down and the basement membrane lifted off the basal cell layer.

uniform shape, and as the attachments fail, the integrity of the basal cell layer diminishes until it is no longer able to maintain the connection to the basement membrane, and separation of the laminae can occur (*see* Fig. 224).

Following MMP activation of the explants, the basal cell layer remained intact and it was the attaching filaments of the hemidesmosomes, between the basement membrane and the basal cell layer, that were broken down (*see* Fig. 225).

The changes in the laminae from horses with experimentally induced laminitis are not as clear cut as this. In carbohydrate (oligofructose)-induced laminitis, both patterns are seen, with a loss of integrity of the basal cell layer as well as loss of the attaching filaments, and because the laminae are under tension in the live horse, the basement membrane itself is damaged as it is pulled away from the basal cells.

Could these Findings Give us a Clue on how Insulin Resistance Plays a Part in Laminitis?

Laminitis induced in normal (non-IR) ponies

and horses by giving very high doses of insulin (hyperinsulinemia) via an intravenous drip develops around thirty hours after the drip is started and worsens while the drip is maintained. Under electron microscopy, the laminar changes found in these horses and ponies are similar to those found in the explants that separated when glucose uptake from the medium was prevented.

Glucose was given, in these studies, to maintain blood glucose levels in the normal (safe) range, so in order to see the effect of this glucose, a further experiment was carried out giving equivalent amounts of glucose without any insulin. This glucose caused the release of increased amounts of insulin from the horse's pancreas to keep blood glucose within the normal range, and resulted in levels of blood insulin that are not uncommonly found in IR horses and ponies. Clinical laminitis did not occur in this experiment, but changes in the laminae were seen when looked at under the microscope, which indicates that the laminitis caused in the first experiments was as a result of the insulin given, and not the glucose.

How Does this Fit into what we Find 'in the Field'?

In insulin-induced laminitis, the very high levels of insulin caused sufficient loss of desmosomes, hemidesmosomes and internal cytoskeleton to cause laminar breakdown and clinical laminitis. However, in most horses that we see 'in the field', the peak level of insulin in the blood, following feeding, is extremely unlikely to reach those levels that occurred in the experimental model, and it is the more minor changes seen in the laminae, caused by lower levels of insulin resulting from the glucose drip, which seem to be much closer to that seen 'in the field'. In this situation, what we would expect, if changes result directly from the effect of insulin, is intermittent damage to occur when the insulin level rises in response to feeding, particularly if the horse has a diet high in sugar (simple sugars and starch).

Intermittent high levels of insulin will affect fewer desmosomes and hemidesmosomes, and less cytoskeleton will be lost than in the high-dose insulin studies. Although in many IR cases this effect is not sufficient to affect the integrity of the attachment to cause lameness, the laminae are in a weaker state than they should be, and may be weak enough to produce the changes in the feet referred to as 'low grade laminitis'.

The Possible Effects of IR

Because laminar separation occurred if glucose uptake from the medium by the basal cells was blocked, my initial thought was that it could be reduced sensitivity of the basal cells to insulin, in IR, that might deprive them of glucose, cause breakdown of their attachments, and result in laminar separation. However, it has been shown that the laminar basal cells are not dependent on insulin for uptake of glucose, so changes in insulin sensitivity has no direct effect on them. Laminar basal cells have been identified as having a high demand for glucose as an energy source, and having a simpler (not insulin-dependent) mechanism for glucose transfer means that if glucose is present in the blood, it can be taken up by the basal cells.

If it is glucose deprivation that causes the loss of the basal cell attachments, then the only way it can come about is if the blood supply to the laminae is affected and glucose is unable to reach the cells. This seems a reasonable suggestion, because many of the problems encountered in human diabetics are due to effects on peripheral blood supply, including high blood pressure and atherosclerosis, which can, in some cases, necessitate amputation of part of a limb. This idea seemed unlikely because, as with the laminar basal cells, glucose

uptake by vascular smooth muscle is insulin-independent and the normal effect of insulin is to dilate blood vessels.

However, experiments using isolated laminar blood vessels appear to indicate that, in IR, the response to insulin is to cause contraction of these vessels rather than dilation. This would account for the observation that there is increased blood flow in the feet early on in the insulin-drip experiments, from vasodilation caused by the insulin, but the continuing effect of high levels of insulin, causing IR to develop, would then result in venoconstriction, which could cause glucose deprivation. Other work has also found abnormal responses to cytokines in laminar blood vessels from cases of laminitis.

Can these Changes Contribute to Laminitis Involving the Different Trigger Factors?

IR and Mechanical Triggers

Regardless of what causes the laminae to separate from the basement membrane, it is the mechanical forces acting on them that pull them apart. Any weakening of the laminae due to IR will make them more liable to mechanical separation. This may be a reason for some cases of 'road founder'.

In 'supporting limb laminitis', constant weight-bearing on the uninjured leg will inevitably limit blood perfusion in the foot, and could be sufficient to cause glucose-deprivation in the laminae. The pain and stress from the initial injury could cause metabolic changes that could further contribute to the weakening of the laminae and to laminar separation.

IR and Metabolic Triggers

The increased corticosteroid levels occurring in PPID and from drug administration cases may exacerbate the effects of IR on the laminae.

In a similar way, the increased cortisol levels and norepinephrine-induced vasoconstriction resulting from 'stress' may worsen IR.

Infectious and Inflammatory Conditions

Laminitis is associated with intestinal conditions where there is damage to the gut wall. This can be due to changes to the gut flora, in carbohydrate overload (CHO) as a result of fermentation of NSCs, or from the proliferation of infectious organisms – for example the intracellular bacterium that causes Potomac horse fever (*neorickettsia risticii*), causing colitis – but it can also occur from restriction of blood flow due to twisting of the gut. In these situations, damage to the gut wall appears to allow some form of 'trigger factor' to escape into the bloodstream, and a similar situation occurs in cases of metritis, when the mucosal lining of the uterus is damaged.

Of these conditions, a lot more is known

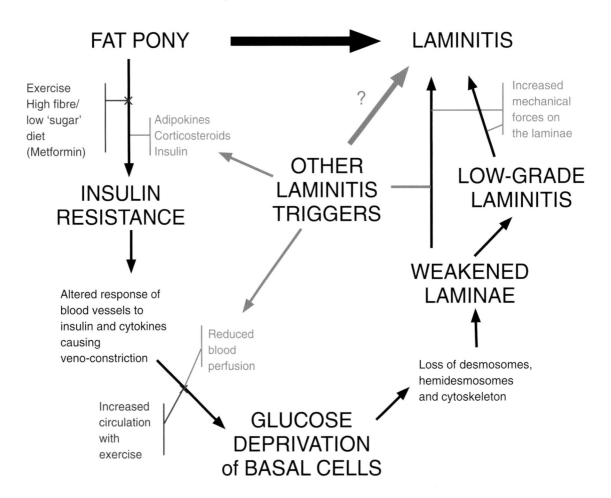

Fig. 226 *A possible explanation for why fat ponies (and fat horses and donkeys) are prone to developing laminitis. The factors in blue (mainly diet and exercise) are positive features, reducing IR and its effects. Those in red are contributory factors to IR or its effects. While 'other laminitis trigger factors' may cause laminitis by some other mechanism, it is likely that many of them also contribute to IR in some way: some will increase adipokine and/or corticosteroid production, while others will affect the blood perfusion of the laminae. They are also more likely to cause clinical laminitis if the laminae are already weakened by IR.*

about the changes that occur in CHO-induced laminitis, because this can be reproduced experimentally. When large amounts of NSC reach the hindgut, there is a rapid and massive proliferation of lactic acid-producing bacteria, which causes the pH of the hindgut contents to fall rapidly. It is only when the pH drops below 6.0 (normally around 6.5), that the gut wall becomes damaged. As a result of the lowered pH, the normal (gram-negative) hindgut bacteria die off, releasing toxins (endotoxin) that contribute to the systemic signs seen in these cases. The clinical signs seen prior to clinical laminitis include inappetence, depression and profuse diarrhoea. Although a form of fructan (oligofructose) is used experimentally, some people doubt that laminitis occurs as a result of fructans in grass. They suggest the following.

- The systemic signs described above are not recognized as symptoms of pasture-related laminitis
- Even when the fructan levels in grass are high, the amount of fructan that a horse or pony eats in a day is less than the dose of fructan used experimentally.
- The fructans in grass are different to those given experimentally and they are ingested over the day, rather than in one large dose. (This point could equally be used in the argument *for* the role of fructan in pasture-related laminitis.)
- The environmental conditions that produce high levels of fructan in cultivated pasture also produce higher levels of simple sugars, and they suggest it is the effect of these simple sugars on IR that causes the laminitis in horses on pasture.

The counter-argument for its involvement is:

- The grasses in cultivated pasture in the UK are very efficient at producing sugars and storing the excess as fructan.

- Particularly in spells of cold sunny weather, the fructan levels in these grasses can be extremely high.
- Studies have demonstrated that, in some circumstances, the daily pasture intake of ponies can be significantly greater than normal, and if this pasture contained high levels of fructan, the amount of fructan ingested over a day would be greater than the dose of fructan used experimentally to induce laminitis (*see* above).

These high levels of 'pasture fructan' taken throughout the day may not produce such dramatic changes, but may still be able to lower the hindgut pH to below the critical pH 6.0 – not enough to cause the obvious systemic effects of inappetence and diarrhoea, but sufficient to produce laminar changes.(This is perhaps a similar result to what occurs when lower limb cryotherapy is used in oligofructose overdose (OFO) experiments, where it is able to prevent clinical laminitis, but some changes in the laminae are seen.)

IR and Carbohydrate Overdose

Whether fructans in grass causes laminitis in non-insulin-resistant horses, or whether IR alone causes pasture-related laminitis, it seems likely that it will be a combination of the two in many cases. To summarize:

- IR horses have a greater appetite and thus are more likely to ingest an increased amount of fructan in a day.
- The conditions that cause pasture fructans to be dangerously high will inevitably be conditions that also result in higher levels of the simple sugars, thus worsening IR and causing further weakening of the laminae.
- If there is weakening of the laminae due to IR, any dose of fructan that causes the pH of the hindgut to fall below 6.0 will make

it more likely that clinical laminitis will occur.

IR and Infectious and Inflammatory Conditions

Very many of these conditions are accompanied by severe systemic effects which will alter the horse's metabolic state, and may either worsen IR to cause laminitis, or trigger separation in laminae that have been weakened by IR. Carbohydrate overload, colitis, strangulation of the intestine, metritis and other infections, and also severe acute rhabdomyolysis (acute breakdown of muscles) all have marked systemic symptoms, but only sometimes trigger laminitis. These systemic changes will be similar to other forms of 'stress', as the body releases corticosteroids to mobilize glucose and break down fat to provide energy.

Other effects are as follows:

- Endotoxins entering the blood through the damaged gut wall affect fat tissue, causing lipolysis to provide energy, stimulating the release of cytokines that are involved in the inflammatory response and have effects on the circulation.
- The body's response is to try to conserve blood flow to the vital structures through the effects of catecholamines, causing vasoconstriction at the 'periphery'.
- Amines produced in the hindgut can gain access through the damaged wall and can contribute to vasoconstriction.
- The changes in the response of blood vessels to vasoactive mediators in IR alter how these factors affect them.
- The overall effect appears to be one of vascular constriction, particularly venoconstriction, which accounts for the bounding pulse found with laminitis.

All these conditions cause laminitis, but not every time, and it may be that those horses

that are already insulin resistant will be more prone to succumbing to it.

When black walnut extract is administered to horses, it does not have the marked systemic effects seen with the conditions described above, but there is evidence of vascular changes by the way that all the limbs swell (a symptom not typically seen with laminitis).

Processes Involved in Laminar Breakdown and Repair

Inflammation

Inflammation is a natural defensive response to a harmful stimulus. The inflammatory process tries to limit the effects of the injurious agent and initiate healing. Inflammatory changes are seen in BWE- and CHO-induced laminitis, but not if induced by insulin. Inflammation could be a response to damage caused by a 'trigger factor', but could be because the attachments to the basement membrane are affected in these cases, rather than the loss of integrity of the basal cell layer that occurs in IR.

In CHO, a similar inflammatory response occurs in the front as in the hind feet; also basement membrane detachment occurs in other organs around the body, as well as in the feet. Because the basement membrane reattaches in these other organs once the 'trigger' has gone, and separation is typically greater in the front feet than the hinds, it seems that the extent of the separation is the consequence of the different mechanical forces in the affected tissues.

MMP Enzymes

MMPs are involved in tissue remodelling in normal physiological processes as well as pathological conditions. It was thought that activation of MMP enzymes by a trigger factor caused the laminae to separate, but it has now been found that basement membrane changes occur prior to any rise in activated MMPs.

White blood cells produce MMP9, which accounts for the increased levels in BWE- and CHO-induced laminitis from the inflammatory response, but it remains in its inactive form. A rise in the tissue enzyme, MMP2, is a feature of CHO, but most of the increase is in the inactive form.

Having been shown not to initiate the laminar separation, the activation of MMP2 may actually be a physiological response in the healing process. MMP activation occurs in skin that has been damaged, breaking down already damaged collagen and allowing the basal cells to migrate and proliferate to speed up the recovery of the wound, and it is possible that this could be their role in laminitis. This would account for the lower levels of MMP found in the laminae in hind feet, where less separation occurs. It may be because the basement membrane is not directly damaged that there is no rise in MMPs in insulin-induced laminitis.

Unfortunately, if activation of the MMPs is a 'healing' response, because the laminae are under tension, detachment of basal cells to allow migration will result in further separation. If this is the case, it would be a strong indication for using cryotherapy, not just for prevention but also as a treatment in infectious and inflammatory conditions where MMP activation occurs.

Increase in Basal Cell Division

Normally there is limited division of the epidermal basal cells of the laminae, but as soon as the laminae are damaged, basal cells start to multiply to repair the injury. In the insulin-induced laminitis experiment, the changes seen under the microscope after fifty to sixty hours were described as 'lamellar lesions normally characteristic of acute and chronic laminitis'.

There was increased basal cell division and lengthening of the laminae, and there were only localized areas of separation of the basal cells from the basement membrane. Progressive weakening of the basal cell layer is likely to produce small areas of breakdown that a localized increase in cell division is able to repair while further areas are breaking down, and if a lot of these small areas of damage are repaired in this way, this process provides an explanation for the lengthening of the laminae that is found in these cases.

In oligofructose overdose experiments, the changes seen in the laminae are a combination of the two types of separation found in the explant experiments (see Figs 224 and 225). With both breakdown of basal cell attachments as well as of the filamentous attachments to the basement membrane, it appears that at least part of the laminar separation is caused by metabolic changes. The significant rise in basal cell division occurring in BWE-induced laminitis could indicate metabolic involvement in this situation too.

IN CONCLUSION

As I pointed out at the start of the chapter, some of what I have written is speculation, combining my interpretation of other peoples' research work with the results of my own studies. Undoubtedly a lot more research will need to be done before the full story is revealed, but even if my theories turn out to be incorrect, I believe the underlying principles are likely to be the same. There seems to be little doubt that if owners ensure that their horses are not allowed to become fat, are regularly exercised, have their feet trimmed regularly, and are fed a suitable, predominantly 'fibre' diet, then the chances of their horse developing laminitis will be vastly reduced.

Abbreviations Used in this Book

A-V shunts Arterio-venous shunts

ACTH Adrenocorticotropic hormone

Bute Phenylbutazone

CDA Coronary band/Dorsal wall Angle

CHO Carbohydrate overload

CT Computed Tomography

DDFT Deep Digital Flexor Tendon

DST Dexamethasone Supression Test

EMS Equine Metabolic Syndrome

ESC Ethanol Soluble Carbohydrates

EVA Ethyl Vinyl Acetate

GLUT Glucose Transport protein

HPA Hoof Pastern Axis

IR Insulin Resistance

MMP Matrixmetallopropinase (enzymes)

MRI Magnetic Resonance Imaging

NSAID Non-Steroidal Anti-Inflammatory Drugs

NSC Non-Structural Carbohydrates

P1 First Phalanx = Proximal Phalanx = Long Pastern Bone

P2 Second Phalanx = Middle Phalanx = Short Pastern Bone

P3 Third Phalanx = Distal Phalanx = Coffin Bone = Pedal Bone

PAD Palmer Angle Determiner

PPID Pituitary Pars Intermedia Disease

SDFT Superficial Digital Flexor Tendon

WSC Water Soluble Carbohydrates

Glossary

Abaxial   turned outwards

Adipo-   related to fat e.g. adipose tissue and adipokine

Amino acids   organic compounds that are the basic 'building blocks' of proteins

Anaerobic   absence of oxygen, e.g. anaerobic bacteria that thrive in places where there is no oxygen

Analgesic   a 'pain-killer' – a drug that relieves pain

Antero-posterior   from front to back

Arterial   relating to arteries

Articular   relating to joints

Axial   turned inwards

Carbohydrate   the range of simple to complex sugars that occur in plants and animals

Caudal   posterior or back of

Caecum   part of the horse's large gut where the breakdown of fibre in the diet occurs

Circumflex   curving around

Collateral   alongside

Commissure   where two structures are joined

Coronary   related to the area of the coronary band at the top of the hoof wall, e.g. coronary corium, coronary papilla

Digital   related to the digit

Distal   further from the body

Dorsal   the front surface

Dorso-palmar   from front to back

Enzymes   proteins that are responsible for speeding up biological reactions

Fibroblasts   Cells that produce collagen and elastin as well as glycoproteins

Hyper-   too much, e.g hyperinsulinaemia is too much insulin in the blood and hyperlipidaemia too much fat in the blood

Hypo-   too little, e.g. hypoglycaemia is too little glucose in the blood

Ischemia   restricted blood supply to tissues

Laminar   relating/pertaining to the laminae

Lateral   the outside of the leg or foot

Medial   the inside of the leg or foot

Median plane   the plane that divides the foot (or leg or body) into two equal parts

Metabolism   the chemical and physical processes that go on in the body that are necessary to maintain life

Neurectomy   cutting the palmar digital nerves to 'permanently' de-sensitize the foot

Neuropathic pain   pain caused by inflammation or disease in nerves that can produce constant pain or a heightened sensitivity to stimuli

Osteo-   relating to bones

Palmar   the back of the leg or foot, e.g. palmar process, palmar surface, palmar digital artery

pH   indicates the acidity or alkalinity of a substance with 7.0 as 'neutral' (pure water). The higher the figure above this the more alkaline and the lower the figure below this the more acidic

Plantar   the back of the hind leg

Plexus   a network of veins

Posterior   the back or towards the back

Protein   biological compounds made up of amino acids. The form and characteristics of each protein is defined by the type and combination of specific amino acids in its make-up. Proteins have many roles in the body; hormones controlling metabolic processes, enzymes affecting chemical reactions, immunoglobulins providing protection against infection and some with mechanical (in muscle) or structural functions

Proud flesh   granulation tissue (healing tissue) that protrudes above the level (is proud to) the surrounding normal tissue

Proximal   closer to the body

Radiopaque   X-rays are unable to pass through, thus will be seen as a white image on radiographs

Sagittal   in the line of the body

Solar   relating to the sole, e.g. solar corium, solar border

Stratum   layer

Trauma   damage caused by an external source

Vascular   relating to blood vessels

Vaso-active   affecting blood vessels, causing them to constrict or to dilate

Venous   relating to the veins

Zona Alba   in this book this refers to the unpigmented stratum medium (some people use it to refer to the 'white line')

-*blasts*   types of cells, e.g. osteoblasts are cells that produce bone or fibroblasts that are cells that produce the structural proteins collagen and elastin

-*cytes*   types of cells, e.g. keratinocytes are keratin-producing cells

-*itis*   disease or inflammation affecting a part of the body e.g. enteritis (gut) pancreatitis (pancreas) lymphangitis (lymphatic system)

-*aemia*   in the blood, e.g toxaemia is toxins in the blood, septicaemia is infection in the blood

References

Chapter 1
'Evolution' presentation by Dr Jeff Thomason, International Hoofcare Summit, 2011.

Chapter 2
Bowker, R.M. 'Contrasting structural morphologies of "good" and "bad" footed horses', 49th Annual Convention, AAEP 2003.

O'Grady, S.E. et al 'Podiatry terminology' *Equine Veterinary Education* Vol 19 (5) pp263–271 (June, 2007).

Leach, D.H. 'The structure and function of the equine hoof wall' (1980), PhD thesis, Department of Veterinary Anatomy, University of Saskatchewan.

Pollitt, C.C. *Anatomy and Physiology of the Inner Hoof Wall* Clinical Techniques in Equine Practice (2004).

Pollitt, C.C. 'Clinical anatomy and physiology of the normal equine foot', *Equine Veterinary Education* Vol 4 (5) pp219–224 (1992).

Pollitt, C.C. 'The anatomy and physiology of the hoof wall', *Equine Veterinary Education* Vol 10 (6) pp318–325 (1998).

'Functional anatomy of the horse's foot' Steven D. In Practice Vol 3 (4) 22-27 1981

Chapter 3
Turner, T.A. 'The use of hoof measurements for the objective assessment of hoof balance' Proc. Am. Assoc. Equine Practnrs. 38, 389–396. (1992).

Chapter 4
Balch, O.K. et al 'Balancing the normal foot: hoof preparation, shoe fit and shoe modification in the performance horse' *Equine Veterinary Education* Vol 9 (3) pp143–154 (Jun 1997).

van Heel, M.C.V. 'Lateralised motor behaviour leads to unevenness in front feet and asymmetry in the athletic performance in young mature Warmbloods' *Equine Veterinary Journal* Vol 42 (5) pp444–450 (Jul 2010).

Heymering, Henry 'The Proper Hoof Angle' *ANVIL Magazine*, Vol. XVI, No. 10 pp19–26 (Oct 1991).

Moleman, M. 'Accuracy of hoof angle measurement devices in comparison with digitally analysed radiographs' *Equine Veterinary Education* Vol 17 (6) pp319–322 (Dec 2005).

Chapter 5
Collins S.N. *et al* 'Radiological anatomy of the donkey's foot: objective characterisation of the normal and laminitic donkey foot', *Equine Veterinary Journal* Vol 43 (4) pp478–486 (Jul 2011).

Hampson, Brian, and Pollitt, Christopher C. 'Improving the Foot Health of the Domestic Horse: The relevance of the feral horse foot model' Rural Industries Research and Development Corporation (RIRDC)

Redden, Dr Ric 'The Wild Horse's Foot' www.nanric.com/thewildhorsesfoot.asp (2001)

Viitanen, M.J. et al 'Effect of foot balance on the intra-articular pressure in the distal interphalangeal joint in vitro' *Equine Veterinary Journal* Vol 35 (2) pp184–9 (Mar 2003).

Chapter 6
Colles, C.M. 'The relationship of frog pressure to heel expansion' *Equine Veterinary Journal* Vol 21 (1) pp6–13 (Jan 1989)

Savoldi, M.T., and Rosenberg, G.F. 'Uniform Sole Thickness' www.americanfarriers.org, Part 1 January/February 2003 p35, Part 2 March/April 2003 p65, Part 3 May/June 2003 p65

Chapter 7
Almgvist, Obel N. and Wilcsells Bottrykeri 'Studies of the histopathology of acute laminitis' Thesis, Uppsala.

Carter, D.W., Renfroe J.B. 'A novel approach to the treatment and prevention of laminitis: Botulinum Toxin Type A for the treatment of laminitis' Equine Vet Sci (2009) 29, 595–600.

Eastman, Timothy G. et al 'Deep Digital Flexor Tenotomy as a Treatment for Chronic Laminitis in Horses: 37 Cases' AAEP Proceedings 9 Vol. 44/1998 265.

van Eps, A.W., and Pollitt, C.C. 'Equine Laminitis: cryotherapy reduces the severity of the acute lesion' *Equine Veterinary Journal* Vol 36 (3) pp255–260 (2004).

van Eps, A.W., and Pollitt, C.C. 'Equine laminitis model: Cryotherapy reduces the severity of lesions evaluated seven days after induction with oligofructose' *Equine Veterinary Journal* Vol 41 (8) 741–746 (2009).

van Eps, A., Collins, S.N. and Pollitt, C.C. 'Supporting limb laminitis' Vet. Clin. Equine 26, 287-302 (2010).

Gantz Tracey, www.thehorse.com/articles/26548/using-force-measurements-to-help-shoe-laminitic-horses, article on farrier Pat Reilly's presentation at the Laminitis Conference, September 2010.

Phipps, L.P. 'Potomac horse fever' *Equine Veterinary Education* Vol 6 (6) pp321–322 (1994).

Pollitt C.C. *Equine Laminitis: a revised pathophysiology* (1999).

Ramsey, G.D. et al 'The effect of hoof angle variations on dorsal lamellar load in the equine hoof' *Equine Veterinary Journal* Vol. 43, pp 536–542 (Sept, 2011).

Chapter 8

Asplin, Katie E. *et al* 'Induction of laminitis by prolonged hyperinsulinaemia in clinically normal ponies' *The Veterinary Journal* 174 pp530–535 (2007).

Boyce, Mary 'Hyperlipidaemia in miniature horses' www.chem.csustan.edu/chem4400/SJBR/99boyce.htm

Dugdale, A.H.A. et al 'Effect of dietary restriction on body condition, composition and welfare of overweight and obese pony mares' *Equine Veterinary Journal* Vol 42 (7) pp600–610 (Oct 2010).

Freestone, J.F. et al 'Improved insulin sensitivity in hyperinsulinaemic ponies through physical conditioning and controlled feed intake' *Equine Veterinary Journal* Vol 24 (3) pp187–190 (May 1992).

Hoffman, R.M. 'Carbohydrate Metabolism in Horses' *Recent Advances in Equine Nutrition* (Aug 2003).

Johnson, P.J., Messer, N.T., and Ganjam, V.K. 'Cushing's syndromes, insulin resistance and endocrinopathic laminitis' *Equine Veterinary Journal* 36, 194–198 (2004).

de Laat, M.A. et al 'Equine laminitis: Induced by 48 h hyperinsulinaemia in Standardbred horses' *Equine Veterinary Journal* Vol 42 (2) pp129–135 (2010)

Rendle, D.I. 'Equine Cushing's: a predisposing factor in infectious disease' *Equine Veterinary Education* Vol 17 (4) pp184–186 (2005).

www.laminitisclinic.org 'Condition scoring 0–5'.

http://umaine.edu/publications/1010e 'Condition scoring 1-9'

www.safergrass.org/articles.html (Many very interesting articles about pasture, diet and feeding)

Chapter 9

Casteliijns, H.H. 'Pathogenesis and treatment of spontaneous quarter cracks – quantifying vertical mobility of the hoof capsule at the heels' *Pferdeheikunde* 5 pp569–576 (2006).

O'Grady, S.E. 'White line disease – an update' *Equine Veterinary Education* Vol 14 (1) pp51–55 (Feb 2002).

O'Grady, S.E., and Casteliijns, H.H. 'Sheared heels and the correlation to spontaneous quarter cracks' *Equine Veterinary Education* Vol 13 (2) 87–89 (2001).

Parks, A.H. 'Equine foot wounds: principles of healing and treatment' *Equine Veterinary Education* Vol 9 (6) pp317–327 (Dec 1997).

Pollitt, C.C. and Daradka, M. 'Hoof wall wound repair' *Equine Veterinary Journal* Vol. 36 (3) 210–215 (2004).

Brandt, S. *et al* 'Consistent detection of papilloma virus in lesions, intact skin and peripheral blood mononuclear cells in horses affected by hoof canker' *Equine Veterinary Journal* Vol 43 (2) pp 202–209 (Mar 2011).

Turner, T.A. 'White line disease' *Equine Veterinary Education* Vol 9 (6) pp313–316 (Dec 1997).

Huntington, Peter, and Pollitt, Chris 'Nutrition and the Equine Foot' www.ker.com/library/advances/303.pdf

Kempson, Susan 'Feeding to improve feet' www.livinglegends.org.au/horse-health/no-foot-no-horse/feeding-to-improve-feet/

la Pierre, K.C. et al 'Lesions associated with atypical black hole seedy toe in the equine foot'.

http://appliedequinepodiatry.org/Articles/Revised%20HKH%20paper%202011.pdf.

Chapter 10

Cripps, P.J.and Eustace, R.A. 'Factors involved in the prognosis of equine laminitis in the UK' *Equine Veterinary Journal* Vol 31 (5) pp433–442 (Sept 1999).

Cripps, P.J.and Eustace, R.A. 'Radiological measurements from the feet of normal horses with relevance to laminitis' *Equine Veterinary Journal* Vol 31 (5) pp 427–432, (Sept 1999).

Dyson, S.J. 'The puzzle of distal interphalangeal joint pain' *Equine Veterinary Education* Vol 10 (3) pp119–125 (1998).

Redden, R.F. 'Equine Podiatry: Radiography of the Equine Foot'.

Redden, R.F 'Interpreting soft tissue parameters and lesions' (2002) www.nanric.com/interpret_lesions.asp

Rucker, Amy DVM, 'Interpreting Venograms: normal or abnormal and artefacts that may be Misinterpreted' Bluegrass Laminitis Symposium Notes January 2004.

Chapter 11

Dyson, S.J. *et al* 'Current concepts of navicular disease' *Equine Veterinary Education* Vol 23 (1) pp27–31 (Jan 2011).

Dyson, S.J. 'Radiological interpretation of the navicular bone' *Equine Veterinary Education* (AE) 20 (5) pp268–280 (2008).

Honnas, Clifford M. et al 'How to surgically access lesions beneath the hoof capsule' www.equipodiatry.com/article_capsule_lesions.htm.

Kidd, J. 'Pedal bone fractures' *Equine Veterinary Education* Vol 23 (6) pp314–323 (Jun 2011).

Milner, P.I 'Diagnosis and management of solar penetrations' *Equine Veterinary Education* Vol 23 (3) pp142–147 (Mar 2011).

Sherlock, C.E., and Mair, T.S. 'The enigma of sidebone as a cause of lameness in the horse' *Equine Veterinary Education* 18 (3) pp136–138 (2006).

Sherlock, C., and Mair, T. 'Osseous cyst-like lesions/subchondral bone cysts of the phalanges' *Equine Veterinary Education* Vol 23 (4) pp191–204 (Apr 2011)

Willemen, M.A. *et al* 'The effect of orthopaedic shoeing on the force exerted by the deep digital flexor tendon on the navicular bone in horses' *Equine Veterinary Journal* Vol 31(1) pp25–30 (Jan 1999).

www.merckvetmanual.com/mvm/index.jsp?cfile=htm/bc/90737.htm 'Ringbone'

Chapter 12

Asplin, K. E. et al 'Glucose transport in the equine hoof' *Equine Veterinary Journal* Vol 43 (2) 196–201 (Mar 2011).

Asplin, K.E. et al 'Histopathology of insulin-induced laminitis in ponies' *Equine Veterinary Journal* Vol 42 (8) pp700–706 (Nov 2010).

Codi, Ovnicek 'Locating internal hoof structure from external markers – Widest part of the foot' *American Farriers Journal* May/June 2010.

Dodson, Dr D. Cuddeford, and Horrell 'The Significance of pH in the hind gut' Third International Conference on Feeding Horses.

Dyson, S.J. *et al* 'An investigation of the relationship between angles and shapes of the hoof capsule and the distal phalanx' *Equine Veterinary Journal* Vol 43 (3) pp295–301 (May 2011).

van Eps, A.W., and Pollitt, C.C. 'Equine laminitis model: Lamellar histopathology seven days after induction with oligofructose' *Equine Veterinary Journal* Vol 41 (8) 735–740 (2009).

Florence, L., and Reilly, P 'Assessing the Strasser Method' *Journal of Equine Veterinary Science* Vol 23 (11) pp502–505 (Nov 2003)

French K.R., and Pollitt, C.C. 'Equine Laminitis: glucose deprivation and MMP activation induce dermo-epidermal separation in vitro' *Equine Veterinary Journal* Vol 36 (3) pp261–266 (2004)

Hampson, Brian, and Pollitt, Christopher C. 'Improving the Foot Health of the Domestic Horse: The relevance of the feral horse foot model' Rural Industries Research and Development Corporation (RIRDC) https://rirdc.infoservices.com.au/items/11-140.

de Laat, M.A. et al 'Continuous intravenous infusion of glucose induces endogenous hyperinsulinaemia and lamellar histopathology in Standardbred horses' *Veterinary Journal* 191(3):317–22 (Mar 2012)

de Laat, M.A. 'The developmental and acute phases of insulin-induced laminitis involve minimal metalloproteinase activity' *Veterinary Immunology and Immunopathology* 140 (2011) 275–281.

Leise, B.S. *et al* 'Hindlimb laminar inflammatory response is similar to that present in forelimbs after carbohydrate overload in horses' *Equine Veterinary Journal* Nov 2012 (pages 633–639).

Longland, Annette C., and Byrd, Bridgett M. 'Pasture Nonstructural Carbohydrates and Equine Laminitis' *The Journal of Nutrition* July 2006, Vol. 136 no. 7 2099S-2102S.

Nourian, A.R. et al 'Equine laminitis: ultrastructural lesions detected 24–30 hours after induction with oligofructose' *Equine Veterinary Journal* Vol 39 (4) 360–364 (2007).

Pass, M.A., *et al* 'Decreased glucose metabolism causes separation of hoof lamellae in vitro: a trigger for laminitis?' *The Equine Hoof – Equine Veterinary Journal* supplement (26) pp133–138 (1998).

Peroni, John F., Marsh, James N. et al 'Predisposition for venoconstriction in the equine laminar dermis: implications in equine laminitis' *Journal of Applied Physiology* 2006 (100) 3 759–763.

Stewart, J.G. 'Strasser's Plastic Sheet' article entered for the Jim Gourlay Prize 2005 and subsequently printed in the *Veterinary Times* Oct 4 2005, Vol 37 No 35.

Venugopal, C.S., Eades, S., Holmes, E.P. and Beadle, R.E. (2011) 'Insulin resistance in equine digital vessel rings: an in vitro model to study vascular dysfunction in equine laminitis' *Equine Veterinary Journal* 43, 744-749.

Visser, M.B., and Pollitt, C.C. 'The timeline of lamellar basement membrane changes during equine laminitis development' *Equine Veterinary Journal* Vol 43 (4) pp471–477 (Jul 2011).

Visser, M.B. and Pollitt, C.C. 'The timeline of metalloprotease events during oligofructose induced equine laminitis development' *Equine Veterinary Journal* 44, 88–93 (2012).

White, J.M. 'Diagnostic accuracy of digital photography and image analysis for the measurement of foot conformation in the horse' *Equine Veterinary Journal* Vol 40 (7) pp623–628 (Nov 2008).

www.fairhillforge.com/Russellarticle.html A comparison of Russell and Duckett methods, originally printed in the *American Farriers Journal* Mar/Apr 1999.

Other websites and studies referred to in the book include the following.

www.3dglasshorse.com ('The Equine Distal Limb' 3D images)

www.marwell.org.uk (Marwell Wildlife)

http://rosirobinson.com (Rosi Robinson – batik artist)

www.horsescience.com (freeze dried hoof specimens)

www.plastinate.com/plastination_pictures/?lang=en (Foot specimens)

www.thedonkeysanctuary.org.uk (The Donkey Sanctuary Sidmouth Devon)

www.metron-imaging.com (Metron)

http://laminitis.org (The Laminitis Trust)

http://thehaypillow.com (The Hay Pillow – 'slow-feeder' hay nets)

http://krosscheck.com (Leverage testing device for lameness examination)

Further Information

The following websites may be of interest to the reader. Some provide access to information obtained following research studies, while others give an individual's opinion reached from their interpretation of research results and from their own experiences. In some cases, their conclusions may differ from mine but, having spoken to many of the authors, I have found that it is often their explanation of how a problem occurs that is different and our advice on how to deal with the problem, in many cases, turns out to be very similar.

Veterinary Surgeons/Veterinarians/Research

www.laminitisresearch.org/ (The Laminitis Research Organization - Director Dr Chris Pollitt) (this web link provides access to a large number of published articles, many of which I refer to in this book)

www.laminitisresearch.org/chrispollitt_publications1.htm

www.coronavistaequinecenter.com/publishedarticles.html (Dr Robert Bowker)

www.nanric.com/dr_redden_notes_archive.asp (Dr Ric Redden)

www.mascalcia.net/eng/articolienglish.htm (Dr Hans Castelijn)

http://equipodiatry.com/podiatry.html (Dr Steve O'Grady)

www.laminitisclinic.org/ (Dr Robert Eustace)

www.animalhealthfoundation.com (Dr Don Walsh 'Waging War on Laminitis')

'Laminitis: recent advances and future directions' The British Equine Veterinary Association Trust – current research articles that can be accessed via www.wileyonlinelibrary.com/journal/evj

Barefoot Trimmers and Farriers

http://hoofrehab.com (Pete Ramey)

www.keithseeley.com (Keith Seeley)

http://appliedequinepodiatry.org (K.C. la Pierre)

www.wildhorseresearch.com (Australian Brumby research)

www.aanhcp.net (AANHCP website)

www.hopeforsoundness.com (Gene Ovnicek)

www.naturalhorsetrim.com (Gretchen Fathauer)

OTHER SOURCES

www.safergrass.org (Katy Watts)

www.epona-institute.org

www.equicast.us

http://pets.groups.yahoo.com/group/EquineCushings/

MAGAZINES

http://hoofcare.com/ (Hoofcare and Lameness Magazine)

http://thehorseshoof.com ('barefoot' magazine)

www.americanfarriers.com (American Farriers Journal)

http://www.americanfarriers.com/pages/
International-Hoof-Care-Summit-Homepage.php
(International Hoofcare Summit in Cincinnati,
organized by the American Farriers Journal –
highly recommended for farriers, trimmers and
vets)

FOOT EQUIPMENT

Epona shoe: www.eponashoe.com

Natural balance shoes and EDSS: www.
hopeforsoundness.com

Equicast: www.equicast.us

Hoof Support Patch (HSP) Fibre-glass supports for
heels: www.vetcell.com

Hoof-filler: www.vettec.com

Imprint shoe: www.imprintshoes.co.uk

Modified ultimates: www.nanric.com

Outlaw shoe: www.outlawshoe.com

Steward clog – see Equicast, equipodiatry or
hopeforsoundness

HORSE HOOF BOOTS

www.easycareinc.com

www.cavallo-inc.com

www.softrideboots.com

www.marquisboot.com

www.hoofwings.com

BIBLIOGRAPHY

Buff, Dr Esco *Limb Length Disparity* (Equine
Anisomelia)

Butler J.A., Colles, C.M., Dyson, S., Kold, S., Poulos
P. *Clinical Radiology of the Horse* (Wiley-Blackwell)

Curtis, S. *Farriery – Foal to Racehorse* (Curtis)

Curtis, S. (ed.) *Corrective Farriery* – Volume 1
(Curtis)

Curtis, S. (ed.) *Corrective Farriery* – Volume 2
(Curtis)

Denoix, Jean-Marie *The Equine Distal Limb* – An
Atlas of Clinical Anatomy and Comparative
Imaging (Manson Publishing)

Hampson, Brian, and Pollitt, Christopher C.
Improving the Foot Health of the Domestic Horse:
Floyd, Andrea, and Mansmann, Richard Equine
Podiatry (W.B. Saunders)

The relevance of the feral horse foot model (RIRDC,
2011)

Jackson, Jaime *The Natural Horse: Foundations for
Natural Horsemanship'* (Star Ridge Publishing,
1992)

Jackson, Jaime *The Natural Trim – Principles and
Practice* (J. Jackson Publishing, 2012)

London, Hickman J. *Farriery: a complete illustrated
guide* (J.A. Allan, 1977)

Pollitt, Christopher C. *Color Atlas of the Horse's Foot*
(Mosby Wolfe)

Pollitt, C. *Equine Laminitis* (RIRDC)

Ramey, Pete *et al Care and Rehabilitation of the
Equine Foot* (Hoof Rehabilitation Publishing LLC)

Sisson and Grossman *The Anatomy of the Domestic
Animals* (W.B. Saunders Co)

Stashak, Ted S. *Adam's Lameness in Horses*
(Williams & Wilkins)

Strasser, Hiltrud *A Lifetime of Soundness* (Sabine
Kells)

Strasser, Hiltrud *Shoeing: a Necessary Evil?* (Sabine
Kells)

Index